Getting into

Dental
School

Getting into guides

Getting into

Dental School

Adam Cross

8th edition

trotman | **t**

Getting into Dental School

This 8th edition published in 2013 by Trotman Publishing, an imprint of Crimson Publishing Limited, Westminster House, Kew Road, Richmond, Surrey TW9 2ND

© Trotman Publishing 2013

Author: Adam Cross
7th edn by Adam Cross published in 2011
6th edn by Steven Piumatti published in 2009
5th edn by James Burnett published in 2007
4th edn by James Burnett & Andrew Long published in 2005
3rd edn by James Burnett & Andrew Long published in 2003
2nd edn by Joe Ruston & James Burnett published in 2000
1st edn by Joe Ruston published in 1996

Editions 1–4 published by Trotman and Co. Ltd

British Library Cataloguing in Publication Data
A catalogue record for this book is available from the British Library.

ISBN 978 1 906041 91 5

Typeset by IDSUK (DataConnection) Ltd
Printed and bound in the UK by Ashford Colour Press, Gosport, Hants

Contents

Contents

About the author

Adam Cross is Vice Principal at the independent college MPW Birmingham and has several years' expertise in helping students gain entry onto competitive undergraduate courses such as dentistry and medicine. In addition to his careers guidance expertise, Adam also helps students with pre-admissions tests such as the UK Clinical Aptitude Test (UKCAT). Adam is a highly regarded teacher of biology and his commitment to pedagogy ensures that he keeps up to date with developments in the fields of science and teaching and learning.

Acknowledgements

I would like to thank all of the individuals who have given their time to provide information to me. In particular I would like to thank Elinor Softley, Manav Gupta, Sarah McGlone, Neelam Hussain, Sameera Mukadam, Samera Altaf and Joanne Lamb, as well as numerous others, for giving me an insight into life as a dental student. I would also like to thank Dr George Mitchell, Dr Tom Fraser and Dr Neva Patel for giving me an insight into the world of dentistry. In addition, I would like to thank the admissions teams from all of the UK dental schools who put up with my countless emails and phone calls, as well as the British Dental Association and the British Dental Health Foundation for providing factual material relating to dental careers. Finally, I would like to thank my wife for her support while I was writing the book.

I would like to emphasise here that although the information in the book has been provided by experts, most of the views expressed are my own, and any mistakes are also mine.

Adam Cross

Introduction

If you have picked up this book, it probably means that you are considering applying to study dentistry and so ultimately want to become a dentist. At this stage of the process, you may be unsure about the details of how to apply, or how best to prepare yourself for an admissions interview. You may have no idea about the type of work experience you will be required to have or the demands of pre-admissions tests. However, the whole purpose of this book is to guide you through the process step by step and ensure that you are prepared to make a successful application and secure your place at university.

This book is divided into the following chapters, which will guide you through each stage of the process.

Chapter 1 focuses on the research you need to do before applying. This is divided between research into universities and potential courses and research into dentistry as a career.

Chapter 2 describes the experiences you will have as an undergraduate and the key elements of the course structure. It then explores options for postgraduate study and the various specialisms that exist.

Chapter 3 includes advice on what to consider when choosing the course you wish to apply to. It looks in particular at what to consider when attending open days and the various academic requirements that the courses have.

Chapter 4 deals with preparing your application to make it as attractive as possible to admissions tutors. It includes advice on the UCAS application procedure and also deals with the UK Clinical Aptitude Test (UKCAT) and how best to prepare for it.

Chapter 5 focuses on the personal statement and how to write it. It looks at the general structure of the statement and the elements that need to be included to make an applicant stand out.

Chapter 6 provides advice on how to prepare for multiple mini interviews (MMIs) and panel interviews. It also gives some examples of the types of questions that you may be asked. It goes on to provide key information on some current dental issues, such as mouth cancer, fluoridation of water and NHS dentistry.

Chapter 7 gives information about international students applying to study dentistry, but also deals with applications from other non-standard applicants, such as mature students, graduates, students who have studied arts A levels, and retake students.

Chapter 8 looks at the options you have on results day and describes the steps that you need to take if you miss the grades or do not hold any offers.

Chapter 9 looks at the financial elements of being a dental student and gives details of fees, student loans and grants across the UK.

Chapter 10 looks at career options in dentistry and the different pathways that a dentist could follow. It also looks at your graduate prospects as a dentist and what typical earnings are.

Finally, in Chapter 11, there are tables providing further information and statistics on dentistry admissions, plus a glossary that can be used to decipher any technical terms you come across.

There are a number of case studies provided throughout the book to support the material being discussed. This information is designed to illustrate the appropriate points and should give you an opportunity to see the issues under consideration demonstrated. Like other books in this series, such as *Getting into Medical School*, this title is designed to be a route map for potential dentists rather than a guide to dentistry as a profession. Further information on issues relating to being a dentist can be found on websites such as the British Dental Association's (the BDA – see www.bda.org), or directly from your own dentist.

Entrance requirements have been given primarily in terms of A level grades throughout the book; information for students who have studied Scottish Highers, the International Baccalaureate (IB) and other qualifications is given in Chapter 3.

What role do dentists have in society?

As you have probably already realised, dentistry involves much more than gazing into people's mouths all day! It is a challenging vocation that requires a wide range of skills to be mastered if you are going to be successful.

So why do people choose to study dentistry? Dental professionals often cite a number of reasons for pursuing dentistry as a career. These include:

- developing your interest in human biology and dental issues
- helping and improving people's well-being and confidence, from the very young to the aged
- being a positive and helpful part of the community
- working with your hands, and being able to demonstrate high levels of manual skill

- working with a wide range of people on a day-to-day basis
- freedom to choose your own patients
- an opportunity to run a business and be your own boss
- flexibility in choosing the length of the working day
- working as part of a team
- status and respect
- money.

Dentistry is definitely not just about teeth, but also about oral health in general. Dentists are increasingly filling a much wider societal role than they once had; in addition to carrying out standard treatments, as oral professionals and health practitioners they look after the well-being of their patients and thus become an important part of any community. Take, for example, the advice that a dentist has to give to patients in relation to good oral health. This may include information and advice on diet, giving up smoking and its possible knock-on effects for general health, and recommendations about courses of treatment.

The British Dental Health Foundation, which is associated with the International Dental Health Foundation, has an interesting website, www. dentalhealth.org, which outlines the variety of issues that dentists have to deal with when treating patients on a daily basis. These include obvious issues such as dental decay and sensitive teeth, but also more wide-ranging themes such as mouth cancer, diet and bad breath. A quick look through this site should give you an insight into the range of skills that a modern dentist needs.

Take, for example, the skills required to deal with patients with special needs. Those with physical disabilities may need assistance to get into the dental chair, while people with learning disabilities may become distressed at the thought of going to the dentist and require extra time to be reassured and appropriately cared for. Some patients may have other special needs, such as communication difficulties or being visually or hearing impaired. People with severe medical problems may also need extra care in order to be treated safely and successfully. A dentist must take account of all these and have the skills to deal with them when providing dental care. A dentist may even have to make different arrangements to meet the needs of the individual, and often home visits will need to be organised. The salaried primary care dental service (SPCDS) in the UK is currently responsible for the treatment of people with special medical or social needs, such as complex medical problems, disabilities or mental health problems, who cannot be treated by general dental practitioners (GDPs). In these cases, some dentists (or community dental officers) are willing to work in a more peripatetic fashion than a full-time surgery environment, and the patient's dentist is responsible for referring them to the local clinic, with any hospital letters and X-rays, to give the community dental officer an idea of the patient's dental history.

Another major aspect of the role that dentists have in society is education. Along with dental nurses they are at the forefront of teaching the public about good dental hygiene. There is a major push for preventive dentistry by the NHS and dentists today. The focus is to promote long-term care of the mouth, teeth, gums and cheeks, and extends, as mentioned earlier, to advice on areas such as diet. Teaching awareness of oral health and hygiene is of paramount importance. Dentists educate patients on caring for their teeth and gums by encouraging them to use fluorides, and to floss and brush. Teaching through direct consultations or via the pamphlets available in surgeries is just one of the ways that this can be achieved, with others including the education of young people in schools, and educating elderly people in nursing homes about keeping dentures clean and viable. Ultimately, the goal of educating the population about oral health and preventive dentistry is to keep the need for major dental treatment to a minimum by maintaining a healthy mouth. As the two major causes of tooth loss are tooth decay and gum disease, the better people prevent or deal with these two problems the more chance they have of keeping their teeth for life. The joint efforts of the dentist, the hygienist and the patient can help to prevent the need for treatment, and so avoid the traditional pattern of fillings and extractions. This is a saving not only to the individual in terms of time and money but also to the community in the long term.

Dentists are often the first to spot medical issues that might otherwise go unnoticed until the problem has worsened. One example of this is oral cancer. There are more than 6,000 new cases of oral cancer each year, and about 1,900 patients die from the disease every year (www.cancerresearchuk.org/cancer-info/cancerstats/types/oral/?a=5441). The role of the dentist is vital in the early diagnosis of the disease and referral for appropriate treatment. Dentists are also the first people to recognise other problems, such as ulcers and cold sores, which could lead to more serious conditions. As with all disease, early recognition is more than half the battle.

Over recent years, the field of cosmetic dentistry has also been an area of rapid growth, with dentists playing an increasing role in providing cosmetic improvements to the public. Not only is this increasing their scope, but it is also a lucrative area in our image-conscious society. Cosmetic dental surgery involves treatments to straighten, lighten, reshape and repair teeth. This can also include veneers, crowns, bridges, tooth-coloured fillings, implants, tooth whitening and correction of bites. For example, as people get older, a face can sag, the chin can stick out and the smile droop if the 'bite' is not corrected – what dentists refer to as 'face collapse'. It can even cause headaches, neck pain and other pains in the body. Thus, there is a need for rectification. Usually, obvious abnormal 'bites' or crooked teeth are fixed early in childhood, but today even mild forms are seen as a problem and more young and mature adults than before are undergoing this type of cosmetic treatment.

What are the necessary attributes of a dentist?

As with any competitive university course and vocation, candidates must be able to demonstrate not only academic ability and the right personal qualities but also commitment if they wish to succeed. Practising dentists, admissions tutors and current students all agree that showing dedication to dentistry is of paramount importance during the application process, during university study and beyond into a dentist's professional life.

It is therefore vital that an applicant to a dentistry course is certain that they want to become a dentist before applying. Wanting to study dentistry because 'you like science' or because 'you want to earn lots of money' is unlikely to be enough to convince an admissions tutor to give you a place. It is also unlikely to be enough to keep you motivated throughout your career.

Dentistry, unlike medicine, offers fewer diverse pathways or opportunities later on in your career. This ultimately means that you must be fully informed about what the career path entails because it is difficult to move effortlessly into something else without some degree of re-specialisation.

In addition to being fully committed to dentistry, a dentist must also be able to demonstrate the following:

- the ability to successfully communicate with patients
- an enjoyment in dealing with people and working in a team
- an ability to reassure patients who are scared or in pain
- a caring and sympathetic nature and immense patience
- a high degree of manual dexterity
- self-motivation
- an enjoyment of science and developments in the field of dentistry
- an excellent memory and an ability to solve problems
- versatility
- mental and physical stamina: remember, a dentist may have to concentrate on a single task for hours
- the ability to multi-task: this is necessary for running a business
- an ability to train and manage people and get the best out of them.

Some of the above qualities will not surprise you. It would be hard to be a successful dentist if you could not bear to be around other people, and unsympathetic dentists end up with few patients. Similarly, if you do not enjoy science, you would be unlikely to gain the necessary grades at A level or pass your exams at university. But often overlooked is the need for manual dexterity; dentistry is probably not a course for you to pursue if you are a particularly clumsy person!

If you believe that you have the qualities listed above, the next step is to investigate what being a dentist is actually like and to find out what a dentist does. In brief, a dentist's job includes tasks such as filling cavities, examining X-rays, applying protective sealant on teeth, extracting teeth, removing decay, and taking measurements and making models for dentures. They also often treat gum disease by performing surgery on patients. As you can see, this is where versatility is needed – and stamina. Patience and empathy are also much-needed attributes, as every day a dentist will be working with both their patients and their staff.

Many people are unaware that dentists are usually self-employed, and the amount of money they earn is directly related to the number of patients they see. Without stamina and self-motivation, you are unlikely, at least at the start of your career, to earn as much as you might hope.

A survey conducted in 2010 revealed that the average student debt of a dental student on graduating was £25,545 (www.bda.org/dentists/policy-campaigns/research/workforce-finance/students-young/student-debt-survey.aspx). With the introduction of £9,000 per year tuition fees in September 2012, there is no doubt that this figure will rise significantly. Many of the students surveyed had multiple debts, including student loans, bank loans, overdrafts, credit cards and debts to parents; the most common types of debt were student and bank loans. Therefore, once qualified, dentists, not surprisingly, need to earn enough not only to support themselves but also to begin paying off their debts.

Are there any downsides to being a dentist?

There are, of course, some negative aspects of dentistry. In its highly informative advice sheet on careers in dentistry (www.bda.org/public/careers-in-dentistry), the BDA outlines some of the factors that prospective dentists should consider when thinking about possible career pathways. Some of the commonly cited downsides relate to issues including stress, the demanding nature of being self-employed, lack of career progression, aggressive or frightened patients, and, last but by no means least, the boredom that can accompany repetitive routine tasks.

If you are worried about any of these, you should talk to your own dentist to see how he or she feels about them. Some dentists will warn students against going into the profession without being aware that dentistry suits people who are prepared to work hard and who enjoy being with other people.

Before looking at the applications and admissions processes in more detail, you may be interested to read what a current dental student had to say about her choice of career thus far. Bear in mind that this could be you in one or two years' time.

Case study 1: Neelam Hussain

Neelam Hussain is a second-year student at Birmingham University.

'Throughout my education I considered pursuing a number of different careers, including dermatology, hairdressing and even TV presenting! I started considering dentistry after I had attended a careers convention at my secondary school. I then spent time researching the details of dentistry as a course and a career and realised how interesting the subject was.

'Following this, I proceeded to organise work experience so that I could get a first-hand feel for what it was like to be a dentist. I found it very difficult to arrange a placement at first, as I had no contacts in my family or among my friends, but after contacting numerous dental practices, I was able to secure two placements. My first was a two-week placement at a general dental practice and my second was a three-day placement at a community dental practice.

'I learnt a great deal from my work experience and this really did confirm for me that I wanted to apply to study dentistry. During my work experience at the general dental practice, I was able to have hands-on experience in developing X-rays and preparing to take impressions for dentures and crowns. Working in a community dental practice demonstrated the vast differences that exist between different types of practice. In particular, I was able to see how dealing with patients suffering from other illnesses affected the approach the dentist took. It also allowed me to see that putting the patient at ease is essential to good-quality dental care.'

Neelam decided to study A level Biology, Chemistry and Mathematics and AS Art and Design and achieved AAAB grades. Following her results, she took up her place at Birmingham University.

'My experience of the course so far has been very exciting. It is very different to school and studying for A levels as there is a lot more work involved. However, the work we undertake is very interesting, which means I don't always see it as work but enjoy doing it! My first year was mainly biology-based, which was great for me as I like biology. However, there was not a massive emphasis on specific dental theory. I did appreciate the small bits of dental work we did such as composite fillings on models of teeth as well as observation sessions at the dental school. So far, it has been fascinating to learn about the anatomy of the body, as well as different bodily systems, which I didn't think I would learn about in dental school. It is not all concentrated on the facial area – it goes much further! In addition to this, the people on the course really do make it appealing and bring out the fun element of the subject.

'To anybody thinking about studying dentistry, I would say definitely do it! The experience I have had so far has been wonderful. Make sure that you do lots of interview preparation, research hot topics related to dentistry and make sure you demonstrate the knowledge you have in your interview.'

1 | What do I need to do before applying?

According to UCAS, in 2011 there were 3,197 applicants for entry into dentistry courses competing for 1,196 places, a ratio of 2.67 applicants per place. The ratio of female to male applicants was about 55:44, and the number of places gained by women was slightly higher than those gained by men, with a success rate of 39% (687 acceptances from 1,761 applications) in comparison with 35% (509 acceptances from 1,436 applications) respectively. In other words, women were, on average, slightly more successful than men in their applications. This might be due to a more mature approach, better preparation and focus and better AS level grades, or it may just be due to chance.

Around 473 of the total number of applicants were from overseas, with 83 being accepted. It is more difficult for your application to be successful if you are an overseas applicant, and the reasons for this are discussed further in Chapter 7.

The 2011 numbers signal a decrease in the number of applications in 2010: with 3,720 applying in 2010 and 3,197 in 2011. This represents a 14% decrease in applications between 2010 and 2011. There are a number of factors that are possibly causing this dip in applicant numbers; probably the most important one being the introduction of £9,000 tuition fees. Despite these short-term fluctuations in numbers, it is clear that there is still an extremely strong demand for places on dental courses, as demonstrated by applications being nearly 10% higher in 2011 compared with 2006.

Prospective dental students should therefore ensure that they are not lulled into a false sense of security; a dip in applications does not mean easier entry! As has always been the case, top grades and thorough preparation are irreplaceable when trying to make a successful application. Table 1 in Chapter 11 (see page 119) gives an indication of the application numbers between 2006 and 2011. Against the backdrop of declining numbers, it is interesting to see that the only group of applicants who increased in number were female international students from outside the EU, showing nearly an 11% increase.

Exploring the options

So what are the steps that you need to take to ensure that you have an excellent chance of being selected for an interview and offered a place?

The first step is to thoroughly research the stages of the application process and the demands of the course and career. This is vital for a number of reasons. You need:

- to see whether dentistry is the right career for you
- to see whether your personal and academic skills are matched to the course
- to find out which universities offer dentistry and to which you want to apply
- to find out the details of courses offered by each university and the one that might best suit you (while the courses may have the same title, their structures can differ)
- to give you ideas and information about possible work experience placements
- to find out what makes an excellent personal statement
- to understand the demands of the interview process and to develop interview skills.

Ideally, your research should start in your AS year (Fifth year in Scotland) or even earlier; the most committed prospective dentists I meet often start their preparation in year 10 or before. Most schools start a programme of UCAS and career prospects-related workshops halfway through the AS year, with the aim being that students should have a clear idea about where they want to apply after the summer holidays. However, you should make your mind up about studying dentistry as soon as possible to give you the maximum amount of time for research and work experience placements.

There are several areas that need to be considered in your research. These can be divided into:

- media research: internet, books, periodicals and specialist magazines
- discussion with professionals
- work experience.

Some suggestions for media research are given below.

Internet

- The UCAS website (www.ucas.com) is very useful for research into degree courses and gives comprehensive details about the entry requirements and course structure at each university.

- Newspaper sites: the *Guardian* (www.guardian.co.uk/education) and *The Times* (www.thetimes.co.uk) provide useful information about university league tables and subject rankings.
- The British Dental Association (www.bda.org) gives information primarily on topical issues for healthcare professionals.
- The British Dental Health Foundation (www.dentalhealth.org) focuses more on raising public awareness of important oral hygiene issues. Both of these websites are useful if you want to gain a wider understanding of current issues.
- www.dentistry.co.uk: this is an online periodical that is very useful for up-to-date information about the field of dentistry.
- University websites: most of the information you will need about applying to a university and about the course can be found on individual universities' websites. These are a treasure trove of information and will help you get a feel for each institution and the nature of the course it is offering.

Books and periodicals

- *HEAP 2014: University Degree Course Offers* by Brian Heap has a short section on dentistry and the universities offering dentistry courses, and gives a good overview of entry requirements.
- University prospectuses: calling universities and asking them to send you their prospectus will help you get a feel for the institution and the course. Note that a number of universities have full prospectuses online.
- Subscribing to magazines such as *The Dentist* will let you find out first hand about issues and developments in dentistry. This would be seen as extracurricular reading and would demonstrate your interest to university admissions panels.

Work experience

Discussing your interest in dentistry with dentists working in the field is an excellent way of gathering first-hand information about the subject. It may be a good idea to start by talking to your own local dentist or any family members or friends who are dentists. Ask them as many questions as you can think of about studying dentistry at university and about the career options for dentists. Make sure you ask about the positives and negatives of the job, as practising dentists are the individuals who are best placed to answer these questions honestly. It would also be worth asking about any interesting current issues in dentistry.

However, by far the best thing you can do to decide whether dentistry is for you is to organise, either by yourself or via your school, some work experience in a practice, where you will be able to work-shadow a dentist. This should answer any questions you may have and will also give you an opportunity to find out what goes on in a dental surgery and some of the responsibilities that a dentist has to fulfil. Remember, gaining relevant work experience is not just a desirable part of your application – for the vast majority of courses it is now a prerequisite; it is unlikely that you will be considered unless you have evidence of this. Even more importantly, work experience is a chance for you to decide whether dentistry is the right career for you. I have seen a number of students who have expressed a desire to be a dentist but then totally changed their minds after a week of shadowing and obser-vation. Conversely, I have also seen many students who have shown increased dedication to pursuing a career in dentistry following work experience.

Most admissions tutors agree that the absolute minimum amount of time that prospective dental students should spend work-shadowing dentists is two weeks; anything less than this and you will be unlikely to appreciate the realities of dentistry as a career. However, as the admis-sions process becomes increasingly competitive, most admissions tutors want you to demonstrate an ongoing commitment to the field of dentistry. This means that you should ideally aim to spend time with several different dentists on a regular basis over a number of months. Simply carrying out the basic two weeks is unlikely to display the required commitment. This fact alone means that preparation for your application to study dentistry needs to start as soon as possible, prefer-ably in your AS year (Fifth year in Scotland) or earlier; if you decide on dentistry as a career only at the start of your A2 year (Sixth year in Scotland), it will leave little or no time to build up a solid portfolio of work experience. In addition to undertaking work experience directly related to dentistry, it is also essential to show evidence of experience or vol-untary work in a care-based environment; for example, a hospital, a children's hospice or a nursing home. This will also help to develop your understanding of the wider world and other clinical environments and strengthen your application.

How to arrange work experience

If you are lucky, your school will have a scheme whereby it can organise some work experience for you. The disadvantage is that you will then be unable to impress the admissions tutors with your dynamism and deter-mination as you will not be able to say that you arranged the work expe-rience yourself. However, even where work experience schemes exist, it is unlikely that they will provide every placement for you, and so at some point you will have to show initiative by making the necessary arrangements. There are two routes that you should try: approaching local dentists, and making use of contacts that your friends or family may have.

In order to approach local dentists about possible work experience, you should first get the names and addresses of local dental practices from a website such as the Yellow Pages (www.yell.co.uk) or the BDA (www.bda.org). You should then write a formal email or letter, and include the name of a referee (that is, someone who can vouch for your interest in dentistry as well as your reliability). Your careers teacher, housemaster/housemistress or form teacher would be ideal as a referee. An example of a suitable letter is given in the box below.

---

52 Boscombe Road
Shufflefield
SH3 2DS

Mr M. Littlewood [you should telephone the practice for the name of one of the dentists]
Sparkling Smile Dental Clinic
17 Poole Crescent
Shufflefield
SH15 3AB

1 October 2013

Dear Mr Littlewood

I am currently in my first year of studying A levels in Biology, Chemistry, Maths and Psychology at Shufflefield School, and I am interested in pursuing a career in dentistry. I was wondering if it would be possible to meet you to discuss what the profession is like and then perhaps spend a week shadowing you or one of your colleagues, so that I can get some first-hand experience.

If you require a reference, please contact my form tutor, Mr Jones. His contact details are as follows:

Mr T. Jones
Shufflefield School
Shufflefield
SH21 2CF

I look forward to hearing from you.

Yours sincerely

Mr Robert Smith

Shadowing dentists is useful for a number of reasons.

- It will help you to decide whether you really want to be a dentist.
- It will demonstrate your commitment to studying dentistry to admissions tutors.
- You may, if you can demonstrate to the dentist that you are serious about dentistry, be able to ask him or her for a reference in the future.

Things to look out for during work experience

Your work experience will provide you with invaluable opportunities to develop your knowledge and understanding of dentistry as a career. It is therefore vital that you pay close attention to what is going on around you so you can get the most from the experience. It is a good idea to carry a notebook and pen so that you can jot down answers to questions you have asked as well as any thoughts or observations relating to your experiences. In addition, it is worth trying to keep a diary of what you have observed as this will be an invaluable resource when it comes to writing a personal statement and attending interviews.

Make sure you are as professional as possible throughout your placements: dress as the dentists dress, and be clean, tidy and reasonably formal. Ask intelligent questions to further your understanding of what is going on. Offer to help the dentist or the receptionists with routine tasks. Show an interest in all that is going on around you, bearing in mind that this might be your job in a few years' time.

During your placements, pay attention to the following aspects of dental practice.

The attributes of a dentist

Dentists need to be much more than dental treatment robots; it is therefore a good idea to keep a note of the range of characteristics the dentist demonstrates on a day-to-day basis as well as the variety of tasks they carry out. This will help provide you with a list of the sort of skills you will need to develop as a dentist and will ultimately help you in developing the knowledge of dentists you will require for a successful interview.

Interactions with patients

A vital part of the dentist's role is to interact with patients to discuss potential treatment routes and to guide and reassure them. Take time to observe how a dentist communicates with patients, particularly those who are anxious about being treated.

The variety of treatments available to patients

Make sure that you know what you are observing during your placement. Ask the dentist or nurse for the technical names of the procedures you see and for information on the materials and equipment used. Ask about the advantages and disadvantages of different types of filling, implant or denture.

Make sure that you are aware not only of the way that damaged teeth are repaired, but also about preventive dentistry, orthodontics and oral hygiene. You should also try to discuss the dentist's role in identifying other problems, such as oral cancer.

The roles of different team members

In any dental setting, there will be a wide range of individuals involved who are vital to the overall functioning of the team. For example, in addition to the dentist there may also be dental nurses, hygienists, receptionists and administrators. Make sure you take time to talk to as many members of the team as possible and ask them about the role they play.

Working as a dentist

Ask the dentist about his or her life. Find out about the hours, the way in which dentists are paid, the demands of the job and the career options. Find out what dentists like about the job and what they dislike.

Ultimately, being observant and asking questions will help you further your understanding of what is required in being a dentist. At the end of each of your placements, you should ask yourself whether this is still a career path that you wish to pursue. If there are any aspects of the work that you dislike, ask yourself whether these would put you off becoming a dentist.

Case study 2: Sarah McGlone

Sarah McGlone is in her third year of studying dentistry at Cardiff University.

'I first decided I wanted to be a dentist when I was seven years old. It sounds strange but teeth have always been the first thing I noticed when meeting new people and that led to my interest in dentistry. As I grew older I took more of a forward approach, going for work experience at a nearby dental practice to see what it was like first hand, and realising that being a dentist not only allows you to help people but it provides you with opportunities to meet people from all walks of life. All aspects of the job appealed to me and I haven't looked back since.

'I initially carried out work experience at the dental practice I attend regularly, and have done since I was a child. My dentist had known for years that it was a career I was interested in and so he made every effort for me to see all aspects of the job, and really helped me come to the conclusion that being a dentist was what I wanted to do in life. During my placement, I realised that dentistry is more complicated and more diverse than I had originally thought – it's not just the teeth that you're interested in as a dentist, it's the entire oral cavity. I also learnt that you can build a strong relationship with patients and that in doing so they will be more inclined to come back for regular check-ups.

'So far, my course has been fantastic! It was overwhelming at first, but I think that's the case with the transition into most university courses – university is very different to sixth form or college. I prefer the style of learning to high school, which was much more of a spoon-feeding technique. The tutors sometimes throw you in at the deep end but they're always a half step behind to make sure you don't sink. Whilst having my first patient was nerve-racking, I always felt supported, and the tutors are always pushing you to work things through yourself before asking for help. I find it has made me a more confident and independent learner. I've also learnt that there is very rarely such a thing as a stupid question and that even if you think you'll sound like a fool it's always best to ask.

'My tips to prospective students: don't leave studying for the UKCAT test to the last minute – it's no fun cramming (trust me!). Do some research into required vaccinations and basic facts about dentistry (i.e. composite and amalgam are often used in restorations) as you may be asked these during interviews. When the time comes for your interview, be relaxed and enthusiastic – you're sussing them out just as much as they are you!'

2| What is it like to study dentistry?

In 2011, the General Dental Council (GDC) carried out a complete review and overhaul of the undergraduate dental curriculum as taught in UK dental schools. The result of this review was that the list of subjects that dental schools had to teach was replaced with a list of expected learning outcomes, which is structured in a similar way to a typical A level subject specification. What this means is that all dental schools will have to ensure that each of the learning outcomes is dealt with over the duration of the course and, as a result, there will be a greater degree of similarity between different universities. However, it is also vital to remember that different dental schools will have different ways of approaching these outcomes, and consequently course structure and teaching approaches may differ greatly; this can ultimately result in massively different experiences for students when studying dentistry. It is vital that prospective students thoroughly research what each dental school has to offer in terms of course structure so that they can truly understand what it will be like to study dentistry at a particular university. This section therefore aims to give you some idea of the key things you will experience as a dental student throughout the duration of your course.

Undergraduate

Studying dentistry in the UK should be a challenging but highly rewarding experience, as the provision at British dental schools is normally first rate. Prospective students should be aware from the outset that attending dental school will require commitment and dedication; ask any current dental student and they will tell you how much hard work is needed to succeed. Undergraduate dental courses last for five years and at the end of their studies students will gain the initials BDS or BChD (the Latin equivalent of BDS) after their name. There is no distinction between these two classifications as both refer to a Bachelor of Dental Surgery; the distinction depends on the dental school that a student has attended.

As outlined above, most of the dental schools have a similar structure in their courses but key differences have begun to emerge in the teaching methodology and delivery of course content. It is therefore important for students to carefully research the details of each course and appreciate the key features. This is obviously vital in selecting an appropriate dental school, submitting a relevant personal statement and preparing for an interview. Many of the dental schools have started to put a greater emphasis on students taking responsibility for their own learning. At Leeds, for example, much emphasis is placed on students undertaking self-directed learning with a focus on clinical dentistry throughout the course.

Universities teach in a range of ways, from traditional large lectures to small tuition groups of around eight students. A number of schools, such as Liverpool and Manchester, have successfully developed courses that have some elements of problem-based learning (PBL) at their core. Many of the dental schools have begun to place a greater responsibility on students to be accountable for their own learning, and prospective students should be aware of terms such as self-directed learning. These approaches are designed to develop an independent and inquisitive approach to learning, using libraries and discussing issues with colleagues to solve problems (as the name suggests). Bristol, by contrast, does not subscribe to the PBL approach, and adopts what it calls a traditional integrated programme of lectures, practicals and seminars supported by opportunities to learn in a more clinical setting. Some courses integrate elements of clinical contact from the first year of the course, while others do not introduce clinical contact until year two or three. At Cardiff, for example, first-year students will have exposure to clinical contact for half a day per week, whereas at Birmingham clinical teaching and patient treatment begin at the end of the second year and start of the third year. As you would expect, all dental schools are committed to using up-to-date technology to help teach the curriculum, and students will notice how keen the various dental schools are to demonstrate this during open days.

Year one

The reason why a dental course lasts five years is that the teaching covers a wide variety of elements. All dental schools will offer one or two years of pre-clinical study that lays the foundation for the rest of the course. This is often taught outside the school and covers some or all of the following themes:

- anatomy
- oral health and disease
- biomedical sciences
- physiology
- biochemistry
- microbiology

- oral biology
- pharmacology.

In addition, students will often cover the effects of anaesthetics and other components common to medicine and dentistry. Furthermore, patient management, communication and team-working skills may also be considered because of the patient-centred nature of the profession.

Years two to five

As the course progresses, the amount of clinical work that you carry out will increase, with most universities offering meaningful clinical contact from the second year, although some have clinical contact in the first year as well. Alongside your clinical work, you will continue with programmes in areas such as oral biology, disease and pathology. You will also learn about the social and psychological aspects of patient care while developing your interpersonal and communication skills.

As the clinical part of the course increases in importance, students often take responsibility for their own patients in the in-house 'mini-practices' or as part of a team comprising students with varied experience (in some schools, this includes training with chair-side assistants, dental technicians and hygienists). During the clinical programme at Birmingham, for example, students are given responsibility for their own patients' treatment in what amounts to their own mini-practice in the dental hospital. Students are also encouraged to participate in practitioner attachment schemes in which they spend time with GDPs, specialist dental units and SPCDS. Time can also be spent at local hospitals to gain experience of accident and emergency, ear, nose and throat, and general surgery. In order to teach the patient care necessary to treat a range of people effectively, many schools are now offering courses in behavioural sciences and the management of pain and anxiety, as well as in the treatment of children, the elderly and disabled people. Clinical students will typically study some of the following courses:

- behavioural science
- dental biomaterials
- dental public health
- dental prosthetics
- haematology
- operative technique and clinical skills
- paediatric dentistry
- restorative dentistry
- oral medicine and surgery
- oral pathology
- oral biochemistry and biology

- orthodontics
- endodontics
- prosthodontics
- periodontics
- nutrition and diet
- medico-legal and ethical aspects of dental practice
- forensic dentistry
- sedation
- oral radiology
- other aspects of the management of pain and anxiety in dentistry.

A small number of students who perform well in the examinations at the end of the second, third or fourth year of study (depending on where you study) may have the opportunity to complete an intercalated BSc, although not all dental schools offer this option. This is normally a one-year project, during which students have the opportunity to investigate a chosen topic in much more depth, producing a written thesis before rejoining the course.

Your final years of study consist of a common core of academic work and clinical dental practice and are designed to consolidate and enhance all of the work and experience from your previous years of study. You will continue to have extensive and varied clinical exposure in a number of settings throughout this time. As you near the end of your clinical course, you may have time to pursue your own elective programme of study – a topic of personal interest, which you research on your own. This elective study may include learning a foreign language and in some cases can involve travel abroad. For example, Cardiff is actively involved in the Erasmus exchange programme and has formal links with institutions in Sweden, the Netherlands, Italy and Turkey, among others. Dundee also has links through the Erasmus programme with universities in Denmark, Finland, France, Germany and Norway. A number of other dental schools also have excellent working links with European universities. This means that under the Erasmus scheme, a limited number of students study at another participating European university and are accredited for the academic work they do there.

At the end of year five, there is the final BDS/BChD professional examination. On successful completion of the course, graduates are competent to carry out most treatments and exercise independent clinical judgement.

Two examples of course outlines are provided in the boxes below to illustrate the common threads and differences between different universities.

Programme structure: King's College London (2013)

The King's dental degree programme, in line with General Dental Council recommendations, incorporates the latest thinking in dental education early clinical exposure, an emphasis on ideas as well as facts, integrated teaching of all subjects with an emphasis on a systems approach, and a dimension of choice of special subjects by the student. The integrated nature of the programme means that basic science teaching will relate to clinical practice and clinical teaching will be underpinned by scientific understanding. You will have contact with patients from the first few weeks of the first year and will be encouraged to assume an appropriate level of responsibility for patient care at an early stage. The programme emphasises whole patient care, which implies consideration of the patient's total dental and medical needs, rather than just the provision of items of treatment. Most of the teaching is carried out in small groups where students and staff get to know each other well. The fact that the Dental Institute is the largest in the country with a total intake (for all programmes) of 164 students brings many advantages, including expertise in all areas of dentistry.

The programme has three main components. The first consists of subjects common to medicine and dentistry, progressing from biomedical sciences, through behavioural sciences, epidemiology, pathology and microbiology to human disease. The second includes oral and dental aspects of the biological sciences leading to an understanding of the diagnosis, prevention and treatment of oral and dental diseases and disorders and the effects of systemic disease on the oral and dental tissues. The third component consists of the clinical and technical aspects of dentistry with the provision of comprehensive oral and dental healthcare for patients of all ages. These components are vertically integrated with a larger proportion of basic sciences at first and a larger clinical component at the end.

Throughout the five years of the programme you will, in addition to acquiring the practical skills necessary to become a dentist, acquire communication skills, personal management skills, information technology skills and an appreciation and analysis of ethical and legal issues in dentistry.

Source: www.kcl.ac.uk/prospectus/undergraduate/details/name/dentistry/alpha/DEF/header_search/

Reprinted with kind permission of King's College London.

Programme structure: University of Liverpool (2013)

The programme consists of three phases. Phase I includes the study of Basic Medical Sciences, which you will study via a problem-based learning (PBL) approach in conjunction with lectures. Clinical Dental Skills are introduced during the Special Dental Component in the second semester. Lectures in Oral Health and interactive tutorials in Communication Skills enhance this phase.

Phase II occupies the second, third and fourth years of this integrated programme in which PBL, lectures, seminars and clinical skills acquisition go hand in hand. A wide range of topics is studied including Oral Sciences and Medicine, Oral Diseases, Medical Emergencies, Law and Ethics alongside the theoretical aspects of the various dental disciplines. Training in the practical skills of dentistry is through the supervised treatment of patients in the Dental Hospital.

Phase III is the final year of study, consolidating theoretical knowledge and clinical experience in preparation for the final examination. In addition to treating patients in the Dental Hospital, students also provide treatment in local dental practices and community clinics, thus facilitating a seamless transition into Foundation Training.

Source: www.liv.ac.uk/study/undergraduate/courses/dental-surgery-bds/overview/

Reprinted with kind permission from School of Dentistry, University of Liverpool

Postgraduate

There are many opportunities for postgraduate study in a variety of dental subjects. It is worth noting, however, that before any form of clinical training can commence (i.e. training involving hands-on contact with patients), dental graduates must register with the GDC. Dental schools and hospitals run a wide range of postgraduate programmes that include further clinical and non-clinical training and research degree programmes. The postgraduate courses offered may be as a diploma, master's degree or doctorate and may take from one to two years, or in a few cases up to five years.

General advice and guidance is available from the Royal College of Surgeons of England (RCS) website (www.rcseng.ac.uk/fds/jcptd). However, the specific information relating to each course is best obtained from the website or prospectus of the individual university; this will provide you with the most detailed, up-to-date information.

At Newcastle University, for example, there are eight taught programmes. These are:

1. Clinical Education
2. Clinical Implant Dentistry
3. Clinical Research
4. Conscious Sedation in Dentistry
5. Dental Hygiene and Therapy
6. Medical Sciences
7. Orthodontics
8. Restorative Dentistry.

Newcastle also offers research training that can lead to the degrees of
MPhil or PhD. The MPhil normally requires 12 months' full-time or
24 months' part-time study; the PhD requires a minimum of 36 months'
full-time study (most students complete this within four years).

Other universities are also able to provide a wide range of postgraduate
options. At King's, for example, there are 16 taught graduate programmes, several of which can be pursued via distance learning.

As you might expect, there are also many openings for carrying
out postgraduate research into related areas of dentistry at these
institutions.

In addition to the more formal postgraduate qualifications, qualified dentists are also required to participate in a specified amount of mandatory
continuous professional development (CPD). This comprises short
courses for qualified dentists who want to develop their knowledge of
the latest methods, equipment and techniques. It is the GDC that spec-
ifies the requirements for CPD for dental professionals. Numerous institutions offer CPD, but there are details of a wide range of activities on
each of the postgraduate deanery websites listed in Chapter 11.

Specialisms

The following sections briefly look at the major specialisations in dentistry
as outlined by the GDC. Information on specialisms can be found at
www.gdc-uk.org/Membersofpublic/Lookforaspecialist.

Special care dentistry

This specialism relates to the improvement of the oral health of adoles-
cents and adults who have some form of impairment or disability.

Oral surgery

Oral surgery is used to correct a wide spectrum of diseases, injuries and defects in the jaw and mouth. This is a slightly more intrusive form of surgery than typical root canal or cavity fillings. It usually requires the use of anaesthetic and therefore patients take longer to recover. Examples of oral surgery include having wisdom teeth removed and getting dental implants.

Orthodontics

Orthodontics is a specialty of dentistry that is centred on the study and treatment of malocclusions (improper bites), which may result in tooth irregularity, out-of-proportion jaw relationships, or both. Orthodontic correction has a very positive effect on facial appearance.

Paediatric dentistry

Paediatric dentistry is the practice and teaching of and research into oral healthcare for children from birth to adolescence. Children are unique in their stages of development, oral disease and oral health needs, which is why paediatric dentistry covers all aspects of their oral healthcare. It aims to improve oral health in children and encourage the highest standards of clinical care.

Endodontics

Endodontics deals with the health, injuries and diseases of the pulp and periradicular region (the tooth root and its surrounding tissue), such as root canal injuries, which can harm the nervous system as well.

Periodontics

Periodontics is the branch of dentistry dealing with the supporting structures of teeth and includes the treatment of patients with severe gum disease.

Prosthodontics

Prosthodontics deals mainly with the replacement of hard and soft tissues using crowns, bridges, dentures and implants. It focuses on treatment planning, rehabilitation and maintenance of the oral function, comfort and appearance.

Restorative dentistry

Restorative dentistry is the study, diagnosis and effective management of diseases of the teeth and their supporting structures. It includes endodontics, periodontics and prosthodontics.

Dental public health

Dental public health is a non-clinical specialty that includes assessment of dental health needs and ensuring that dental services meet those needs. It is mainly concerned with improving the dental health of a population rather than that of individuals and involves working in primary care trusts, government offices and strategic health authorities. There are a few such academic posts in universities and in the Department of Health.

Oral medicine

This is concerned with the diagnosis and non-surgical management of medical pathology affecting the oral area, jaw and face. Many oral medicine specialists have dual qualifications, with both medical and dental degrees. The main aspects of oral medicine are clinical care, research and undergraduate and postgraduate teaching.

Oral microbiology

This is the study of the diverse and complex microbial community in the mouth and is carried out by laboratory-based professionals. The primary role of an oral microbiologist is to diagnose bacterial and fungal infections in the head and mouth.

Oral pathology

Oral pathology is the branch of dentistry concerned with diseases of oral structures, including soft tissues, teeth, jaws and salivary glands. It is a science that investigates the causes, processes and effects of these diseases. The practice of oral pathology includes research into and diagnosis of diseases using clinical, radiographic and biochemical means.

Dental and maxillofacial radiology

Dental and maxillofacial radiology involves a combination of radiology and dentistry. It is mainly concerned with using and understanding the diagnostic imaging modalities that are used in dentistry.

3 | Choosing your course

To gain a place at dental school, you have to submit a UCAS application. However, before you do so it is essential that you have thoroughly researched the application process and the demands of dentistry as a profession. Most people have little understanding of the tasks and challenges that a dentist faces on a day-to-day basis and the career pathways available after graduation. It is therefore vital that you are aware both of what being a dentist entails and of the details of the application process before you consider applying to study dentistry. This will ultimately mean that whatever choice you make it will be a well-informed one.

Choice of school

Once you have completed your work experience and are sure that you want to be a dentist, you need to research your choice of dental school.

There are various factors that you should take into account:

- the type and structure of the course
- the academic requirements
- whether the dental school requires you to sit the UKCAT
- the location and type of university
- whether the dental school is part of a large university or is a stand-alone medical and dental school.

The next step is to get hold of the prospectuses. All universities offer detailed information on their websites, with some having complete online prospectuses, so it is well worth spending some time looking here initially. If you cannot find the information you are looking for, it may be worth looking at a hard-copy prospectus. These can be obtained by calling the dental schools; they will send you copies free of charge. In Chapter 11, there is a list of major dental organisations in the UK that you can contact for further information, and a list of the 15 dental schools and their contact details. You can approach the university with any questions relating to admissions or to the course itself. What you must remember is that information on websites and in prospectuses is always changing, so if you're in doubt it is always best to call the university and speak to someone to get the most up-to-date information.

Apart from talking to current or former dental students or careers advisers, there are a number of other sources of information that will help you in making your choice. There are various independent league tables of dental schools, ranked by a total score that combines several assessment categories, including teaching scores, student–staff ratios and job prospects. *The Guardian University Guide 2013* (www.guardian.co.uk/education/universityguide) placed Queen's Belfast first, followed by Glasgow, King's, Aberdeen, Liverpool and Manchester, while *The Complete University Guide* (www.thecompleteuniversityguide.co.uk) placed Glasgow first, followed by King's, Manchester, Bristol and Queen's.

Of course, there is no such thing as a bad dental school in the UK, and league tables tell you only a small part of the whole story. They are based on a range of variables and this is why there is a discrepancy between the two tables mentioned above. Remember that league tables are only a guide – they are no substitute for visiting the dental schools, looking at the course content in detail, reading the prospectuses and speaking to those involved with the course.

Open days

Once you have narrowed down the number of dental schools you like to, say, six or seven, you should try to visit them to get a better idea of what studying there will be like. Details of open days can be found on the websites of each university, but sites such as www.opendays.com show details of all open days throughout the year. If you are unable to attend one of the planned open days, it is worth calling the university to see if there are any suitable times when you may be able to look round. Failing this, there is nothing stopping you visiting the university independently to have a casual look around, although it is unlikely that you will be able to see the dental school on a visit like this. Do not simply select a dental school because someone has told you that it has a good reputation or that it has a higher number of places available. You will be spending the next five years of your life at one of them, and if you do not like the place you are unlikely to last the course.

When attending a university open day, there are a number of points to consider that will give you a better idea of whether the course is for you or not. You should start by considering the university itself – think about the following points:

- location of the university and distance from home: some students prefer to live at home or be very close to home, while others like to get as far away as possible
- campus or city university: again, students seem to have strong preferences about the type of university they study at; some prefer to

be in the middle of a big city while others like to be situated on a rural campus, and visiting the university is the only way to get a true feel for its character
- size of the university
- number of students at the university.

When you take time to visit a university you will automatically get an idea about these points. From this you should consider whether it is the sort of place where you would like to study. I have worked with many students who think they would like to go to a particular university and then totally change their mind about it after taking the time to visit.

In terms of the particulars of the course, it is vital to visit the dental school itself so that you can listen to any talks being given by the admissions tutors and get a feel for what the department is like. A number of universities may ask you to book a place on the dental admissions talk as there are often limited spaces, so ensure you have looked into this well before you go to the open day. In addition to any general talks being given, you may wish to talk one to one with a representative from the department to ask specific questions. If this is the case, try to have questions prepared so that you can get the most out of this time.

Academic requirements

In addition to the grades they require at A level, all of the dental schools specify the minimum grades that they want at GCSE as well. This varies from dental school to dental school, but having at least five A or A* grades, with at least B grades in science subjects, English and Mathematics is a significant advantage. There are some differences in requirements, so it is worth checking what each university is looking for. If your grades fall below these requirements, there is little or no point in applying to that particular course; university admissions tutors often comment on how many applicants they immediately reject because they do not meet the published requirements. If you have genuine extenuating circumstances that explain why you have underachieved (due to illness, family disruption, etc.), your referee will need to comment on these and/or on why they expect your A level performance to be better than your GCSE grades indicate.

In addition to specifying A level grades, some dental schools will ask for a minimum grade in the AS level subjects you have studied. At the moment, some specify that this must be an A grade, others a B, and others do not require an AS subject. Even more important is the fact that AS levels contribute 50% to the total A level score, and poor AS level grades will make it difficult, if not impossible, to achieve the required A grades at A level. AS level grades also give admissions tutors more information to go on than GCSE grades and A level predictions alone, since the AS grades will be published in the August preceding your UCAS application. For the student, this means that the first year of A levels is just as important as the second. The typical subject and entry grade requirements for each of the dental schools are shown in Table 2 in Chapter 11. Also included in this table are details of GCSE and AS grade and subject requirements.

In the past, a number of dental schools accepted A level students who had not achieved the required grades the first time. Unfortunately, due to the competitive nature of dentistry courses, it is now increasingly unlikely that applications from retake students will have a chance of being successful. There are a few courses that will still consider retake applications, but these usually have fairly strict criteria attached. Take Glasgow for example, where retake students can apply, but only if they have already applied, have received a conditional offer and then have missed it by a narrow margin. Obviously, if there have been genuine extenuating circumstances that have caused you to underachieve and you have evidence of this, then it is worth talking to each university to see if they will consider your application. Table 2 in Chapter 11 gives further information on this and shows which dental schools consider students who have not achieved the minimum grades at their first attempt.

Another issue to be considered is the introduction of the A* grade at A level, as first awarded in August 2010. For entry in 2013, there are no dentistry courses that have made A* grades a part of their offers, and so at the moment there is no requirement to reach this level; however, it is probable that over the next few years offers for dentistry may include at least one A* grade.

Other qualifications

If you are not studying A levels, you should check with each dental school about their requirements. The list below offers a rough indication of what they might ask for.

- **Scottish Highers:** AAAAB–AAAAA at Higher level and two or three subjects at Advanced Higher. Higher level Chemistry and Biology are usually required. The majority of universities require at least two Advanced Highers, usually Chemistry and Biology at grades AB–AA.
- **International Baccalaureate:** 6, 6, 6–6, 6, 7 and 35–37 points overall. Chemistry and Biology should be taken at Higher level, with passes in English and Mathematics at Standard level.
- **European Baccalaureate:** 80%–85% overall, with at least 80% in each science option. Chemistry and another science should be taken as full options.

- **Cambridge Pre-U:** most universities will accept Cambridge Pre-U qualifications with D3, D3, M2–D3, D3, D3 in the principal subjects. Biology and Chemistry will usually be required as two of the principal subjects.
- **Advanced diploma:** most universities do not accept the diploma for entry into dentistry; however, there are a few universities that will consider it alongside other qualifications. In these cases, it is best to contact the university directly to discuss entry requirements.
- **BTEC National Diploma:** some universities are happy to accept this with three Distinctions; however, most universities do not. Once again, it is best to contact the individual universities to discuss their entry requirements.

You will need to check with each university about their specific entry requirements as there is always some variation in their demands.

Non-dental choices

There are five spaces on the UCAS application, but only four of these can be used to select dentistry courses. Make sure you enter dentistry in all of the four spaces. The remaining space can either be left blank or filled with another course choice. Each university that you apply to will not see the other choices you have made and so you will not be discriminated against because of where else you have applied or what you have entered as your fifth choice. When filling in the final space, you must remember that it will have no impact on your other choices; however, you must also remember that you can write only one personal statement, which is likely to be largely irrelevant in relation to the other subject. So, for example, imagine you applied to four dental schools and then used your fifth space to apply for history. The dental schools you have chosen will not see that you have put history as your fifth choice and so this will not affect their judgement about your commitment to dentistry. However, the history admissions team will see from your personal statement that you are totally committed to dentistry and so are unlikely to make you an offer. In light of this, there are some subjects that are more appropriate to put as your fifth choice, such as biomedical science, and you have a much greater chance of receiving an offer for one of these alongside an offer for dentistry. It can also provide you with another option to follow if you do not secure entry onto a dentistry course or do not achieve the necessary grades, keeping the door open for later graduate entry.

If you do decide to put another science-related course as your fifth choice, you still cannot make your personal statement relevant to more than one subject; keep it entirely focused on dentistry. Any attempt to make it attractive to a number of different admissions tutors in different subjects will adversely affect your chances of making a successful application to dentistry.

When thinking about which career to pursue, some students consider both dentistry and medicine at some point. If you consider applying for some dentistry and some medicine courses alongside each other, then you are less likely to be successful in securing a place on either course. You should instead decide on one course and put your full effort into preparing a strong application for it, rather than splitting your focus.

4 | The UCAS application

Navigating your way through the UCAS application process can be daunting and can seem like an impossible task. In this chapter the process has been broken down into manageable chunks.

UCAS Apply

When you apply for UK universities, you do so using the UCAS system Apply. The online UCAS form is accessed through the UCAS website (www.ucas.com). You register online either through your school or college, or as a private individual. Some of the information that you provide on the form is factual, such as where you live, where you have studied, what academic qualifications you have, details of examinations that you are going to take, and which university courses you are applying for. The final section on the form is the personal statement, where you write about why you want to study dentistry, and about yourself. We look at the personal statement in more detail in Chapter 5.

Once your form is complete, it is then accessed by the person who will write your reference; they then check it, add the reference and send it to UCAS. After that, you can keep track of the responses from the universities using the online Track facility.

When to submit your UCAS application

The closing date for receipt of the application by UCAS is 15 October. However, you must remember that this is the deadline by which the form is required by UCAS and so your school or college will most likely have an earlier deadline so they can get your reference written. This will probably be around two weeks earlier. Late applications are accepted by UCAS, but the dental schools are not obliged to consider them; because of the pressure on places, it is unlikely that late applications will be considered. Although you can submit your application at any time between the beginning of September and the October deadline, most admissions tutors agree that the earlier the application is submitted, the better your chance of being called for interview.

The safest bet for getting your application completed and sent as soon as possible is to make a start on it in your AS year. Start researching the different universities and the different courses as soon as possible and then begin writing your personal statement and get feedback on it. Ultimately, you want to be in a position where you have a final draft of your personal statement and all of your choices sorted by the beginning of the September term in your A2 year.

The reference

As well as your GCSE results, personal statement and predicted grades, the admissions team will take into account your academic reference. This is where your headmaster or headmistress, housemaster or housemistress or head of sixth form writes about what an outstanding person you are, how you are the life and soul of the school, how you are on target for three A grades at A level, and why you will become an outstanding dentist. For him or her to say this, of course, it has to be true. The referee is expected to be as honest as possible, and to try to accurately assess your character and potential. You may believe that you have all of the qualities – academic and personal – necessary in a dentist, but unless you have demonstrated these to your teachers, they will be unable to support your application.

Ideally, your efforts to impress them will have begun at the start of the sixth form (or preferably before this); you will have become involved in school activities, while at the same time working hard on your A level subjects and developing strong interpersonal skills, demonstrated by your interactions with staff and students. If you do not feel as though you have done this, don't worry, because it is never too late. Some people mature later than others, so if this does not sound like you, start to make efforts to get involved in the wider life of your school or college, as this will help provide evidence for the people who will contribute to your reference.

As part of the reference, your referee will need to predict the grades that you are likely to achieve. As Table 2 in Chapter 11 (see page 120) shows, the minimum requirement for entry is AAB. If your predicted grades are lower than this, it is unlikely that you will be considered. Talk to your teachers and find out whether you are on target for these grades. If not, you need to do one or all of the following:

- work harder or more effectively, and make sure that your teachers notice that you are doing so
- get some extra help either at school or outside: for instance, an Easter revision course
- delay submitting your UCAS application until you have your A level results.

UKCAT

A number of dental schools now require applicants to sit the pre-admissions test known as the UKCAT (the UK Clinical Aptitude Test) before they apply. This test is designed to help discriminate between the many highly qualified applicants who apply for dentistry courses each year. It is important to note that the UKCAT is **not** based on science content from your A level science subjects, but on assessing your skills and attributes.

Dental schools currently requiring the test are Aberdeen, Cardiff, Dundee, Glasgow, King's, Manchester, Newcastle, Queen Mary, Queen's University Belfast and Sheffield.

Registration for the UKCAT usually opens in early May of the year you submit your UCAS form and closes near the end of September. Testing then starts at the beginning of July and finishes at the start of October. It is vital to consult the UKCAT website (www.ukcat.ac.uk) for the exact registration and testing dates for the year you are applying, so that you know precisely what you need to do and when.

The first step is to register on the UKCAT website. You will be asked to select the test centre where you wish to sit the test and then the date and time. Registration opens in May and you should try to register as early as possible in order to get your preferred date and location; there are a number of students each year who have to travel great distances to find a test centre that still has spaces. It is worth taking the test as soon as possible so that you can make an informed decision about which universities to apply to. For example, if you apply only to universities that use the UKCAT and then you underperform in the test, it may reduce your chances of making a successful application. A much better route is to take the UKCAT before you finalise your choices; this will mean you can make a fully informed choice about which universities to apply to.

The cost for those who took the test in 2012 was £65 for candidates taking the test in the EU before 31 August and £100 for other candidates. Between 1 September and 5 October 2012, the cost was £80 for candidates taking the UKCAT in the EU. There are some bursaries available to students who may struggle to meet the cost of the test; these can be applied for through the UKCAT website.

The test itself is sat at an external centre in the location you have chosen. You should aim to arrive at least 15 minutes before your test time, remembering to take a printout of the email confirming your registration and photographic ID. It is important to remember that you must arrive on time for the slot you have booked; if you fail to do so, you will simply not be able to take the test and will have to rebook for a later date and pay the test fee again. The test lasts for two hours and consists of the following five sections:

1. verbal reasoning
2. quantitative reasoning
3. abstract reasoning
4. decision analysis
5. situational judgement test.

While it is not possible to revise for the UKCAT, students find that the more practice they have had on UKCAT-style questions, the better prepared they feel and the better they perform. The UKCAT website is an invaluable source of information; there is an official guide to the test and a number of practice tests. There are also numerous books available that offer hints, tips and practice questions; it is worth flicking through the various titles in a bookshop to see which is best suited to your needs.

The structure and layout of each section is described below.

1. Verbal reasoning

This section is 22 minutes long and contains 44 questions. The UKCAT website says that this section 'assesses candidates' ability to think logically about written information and to arrive at a reasoned conclusion'. You will be presented a short passage of text (an example is given in Figure 1) and given four statements relating to each passage.

UKCAT Practice Test 3 (Short Version)

In digital recording, the analogue sound that we hear needs to be translated into a series of numbers ('0' or '1'). These numbers represent the changes in air pressure over time that makes up the sound, though we cannot directly 'hear' these numbers as sound.

Digital recordings are made by sending the original analogue sound to an 'analogue to digital converter' (ADC). This converter changes the analogue signal into a series of binary numbers. These numbers are then usually stored on a computer or a compact disc. During playback, the digital sound information is read and sent to a 'digital to analogue converter' (DAC) which changes the sound into an analogue signal that is reproduced by devices such as a loudspeaker or headphones.

Figure 1 Sample UKCAT verbal reasoning passage

For each statement, you must answer 'true', 'false' or 'can't tell' based on the information you are given in the passage (see Figure 2).

A loudspeaker is able to produce an analogue signal.

A. True

B. False

C. Can't tell

Figure 2 Sample UKCAT verbal reasoning question

There are 11 passages in this section, giving 44 questions in total.

2. Quantitative reasoning

This section is 23 minutes long and contains 36 questions. The UKCAT website says that it 'assesses candidates' ability to solve numerical problems'.

In this section, you will be presented with tables, charts and/or graphs and then be asked to answer related questions. Each question has five possible answers to choose from, as shown in Figures 3 and 4.

A distribution centre serves stores within a 50-mile radius. The table below shows how far each store is from the distribution centre.

Distance from distribution centre	Number of stores
10 miles or less	3
11 to 20 miles	15
21 to 30 miles	26
31 to 40 miles	20
41 to 50 miles	16

Figure 3 Sample UKCAT numerical data table

How many stores does the distribution centre serve?

A. 60

B. 70

C. 80

D. 90

E. Can't tell

Figure 4 Sample UKCAT numerical data table question

3. Abstract reasoning

This section is 16 minutes long and contains 65 questions. The UKCAT website says that it 'assesses candidates' ability to infer relationships from information by convergent and divergent thinking'.

In this section you will be presented with two sets of shapes, set A and set B, as in Figure 5.

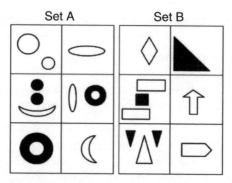

Figure 5 Sample UKCAT shape sets

For each pair of set A and set B, you will be presented with five test shapes, as in Figure 6.

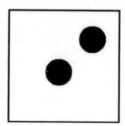

A. Set A

B. Set B

C. Neither

Figure 6 Sample UKCAT test shapes

With each shape, you have to decide whether it belongs to set A, to set B or to neither. There are 13 sets of A and B, giving 65 questions in total.

4. Decision analysis

This section is 32 minutes long and contains 26 items. The UKCAT website says that it 'assesses candidates' ability to deal with various forms of information, to infer relationships, to make informed judgements, and to decide on an appropriate response in situations of complexity and ambiguity'.

In this section you will be presented with a table of codes, as, for example, in Figure 7.

Additional codes

Operators General Rules	Specific Info Basic Codes	Complex Info Additional Information	Reactions/ Outcomes/ Emotions
A = positive	1 = personal	101 = speed	201 = hurt
B = increase	2 = people	102 = injury	202 = excited
C = opposite	3 = air	103 = danger	203 = worried
D = cold	4 = fire	104 = fun	204 = angry
E = fast	5 = water	105 = carry	205 = surprise
F = generalise	6 = earth	106 = empty	
G = combine	7 = sun		
	8 = moon		
	9 = dwelling		
	10 = move		
	11 = today		
	12 = light		
	13 = bag		
	14 = look		

Figure 7 Sample UKCAT decision analysis code table

You will then be presented with 26 questions relating to this table that will require you to decode or encode information or decide on the most appropriate words to add to the table of codes. Each question will have four or five possible answer choices, as shown in Figure 8, for example.

What is the best interpretation of the following coded message:

11, 12, 7

A. Today it is bright and sunny

B. The light from the sun is brighter than usual

C. Today the sun came up

D. Today the sun's rays have a strange hue

E. The sun is floating in the sky

Figure 8 Sample UKCAT decision analysis answer choices

All sample UKCAT questions reprinted with kind permission of UKCAT and Pearson VUE.

5. Situational judgement test

This section is 27 minutes long and can contain up to 60 questions. The UKCAT website says that it 'assesses judgement regarding situations encountered in the workplace'.

Currently, the responses from this section of the test are not used in the selection process and do not contribute to your overall score.

The biggest challenge you will face while taking the test is lack of time because there are so many questions to answer in such a short period. It is vital for you to use the practice tests to get a feel for what it is like to be in a time-pressured situation and to understand how long you can spend on each question in each section.

Deferred entry

Some admissions tutors are happy to consider students who take a gap year; however, if you are considering following this route, you need to make sure that you are going to use the time constructively. A year spent watching daytime TV is not going to impress anybody, whereas independent travelling, charity or voluntary work either at home or abroad, work experience or a responsible job will all indicate that you have used the time to develop independence and maturity.

Having a job during your gap year in somewhere like a shop or a bar may seem like a good idea and is certainly better than sitting around doing nothing all the time; however, if you wish to demonstrate your ongoing commitment to pursuing dentistry as a career, then you should concentrate on getting further experience in a job or placement directly related to the field.

You can either apply for deferred entry when you submit your UCAS application, in which case you need to outline your plans clearly in your personal statement, or apply in September following the publication of your A level results. If you expect to be predicted the right grades, and the feedback from your school or college is that you will be given a good reference, you should apply for deferred entry. On the other hand, if you are advised by your referee that you are unlikely to be considered, you should give yourself more time to work with your referees by waiting until you have your A level results.

Dental timeline

Figure 9 on the next page shows what you will need to be aware of over the course of your A level studies and gives an overview of the timings of some of the various tasks that you should plan for if you are to maximise your chances of gaining entry into a dental school.

As you can see, your main task in your AS year is to start researching your courses and options, organising and carrying out work experience and then preparing your personal statement. The summer between your AS and A2 years should be used to continue building your work experience as well as registering and preparing for the UKCAT. In the second year you must hit the ground running, because the UKCAT and your UCAS application must be finished by early October. At the same time, you must also ensure that you stay on top of your studies so you maximise your chances of achieving the A grades you will need, and you should also start preparing for interview and practising your interview skills. Once your final exams are finished at the end of the year, it is simply a matter of waiting for your results so you can see whether you have secured a place.

Figure 9 Timeline to guide your application to study dentistry

5 | Personal statement

As has been previously stated, the demand for dentistry courses is still extremely high even when taking into account the recent dip in applicant numbers. So what exactly is the impact of sustained high demand for places on dentistry courses?

Almost certainly, the grades necessary for entry into dental school will continue to rise, and, in order to differentiate between applicants, universities will set very high entry requirements. In the late 1990s, when application numbers were lower, candidates often received BBC offers, whereas now the standard offer is AAA. At some point in the future, a standard offer is likely to include at least one A* at A level as well.

Your application is likely to be received by the university and considered along with many others at the same time. On average, a dental school may receive around 700 applications and have to select around 250 to 300 to be called for interview. Of those who apply, there will be some who are automatically rejected as they do not fulfil all the entry criteria; for example, not meeting the GCSE grade requirements. Following this, it is down to the admissions team to try to select whom to interview from the remaining candidates. Many of the applicants who are still being considered at this stage will have excellent GCSE profiles, outstanding predicted A level grades and a strong UKCAT performance. So how do the selectors make their choices?

One of the most important factors at this stage of selection is the personal statement. If this is badly worded, uninteresting or lacking in the things that the selector feels are important, it will be put on the 'reject without interview' pile. Ultimately, this means that the more thought that you give to your UCAS application and personal statement, the better they will be and the greater your chance of being offered a conditional place or being asked to come in for an interview. Remember that the selectors will not know about the things that you have forgotten to say: they can get an impression of you only from what is in the application. I have come across many good students who never secured an interview simply because they did not thoroughly plan and prepare their personal statement.

Note that only a small proportion of applicants will be interviewed, so while it's important to prepare for the interview it's vital that you make your personal statement as strong as it possibly can be. The number of those interviewed depends on the university and can fluctuate widely. Tables 2, 3 and 4 in Chapter 11 provide an outline of the numbers of students that dental schools interview and typical interview policies. For example, in 2011 Liverpool interviewed around 46% of those who applied, which meant approximately 450 interviews out of 970 applications.

The following sections will tell you more about what the selectors are looking for in a personal statement, and how you can avoid common mistakes.

Personal statement basics

When constructing your personal statement, there are several important things that you need to consider. First, your personal statement needs to be no more than 47 lines or 4,000 characters, including spaces; this is a strict limit and so you need to ensure that you are as close to this as possible. You must then consider the key themes of your personal statement, which are:

- why you want to be a dentist
- what your academic interests are and how these have furthered your desire to pursue dentistry
- what you have done to investigate the profession
- what you have done to develop the skills needed to become a dentist
- why you are the right person for their dental school and their particular dentistry course.

The personal statement is your opportunity to demonstrate to the selectors that you are fully committed to studying dentistry and have the right motivation and personal qualities to do so successfully. A typical personal statement takes time and effort to get right: don't expect perfection after one draft. At each stage of the process you should take time to read through your statement, and ask yourself the question: 'Does it sound like me?' If not, redraft it. You should also take the time to get your academic advisers or teachers to give you feedback at each stage; this will ensure you stay on the right track.

Sections of the personal statement

Why dentistry?

This should be your first section and will outline to the admissions tutors your motivation for wanting to study dentistry. A high proportion of UCAS applications contain stock phrases such as: 'From an early age I have wanted to be a dentist because it is the only career that combines my love of science with the chance to work with people.' Not only do admissions tutors get bored with reading such statements, remarks like these are also clearly untrue: if you think about it, there are many careers that combine science and working with people, including teaching, pharmacy, physiotherapy and nursing. Nevertheless, the basic idea of this sentence may well apply to you. If so, you need to personalise it. You could mention an incident that first got you interested in dentistry – a visit to your own dentist, a conversation with a family friend or a talk or lesson at school, for instance. You could write about your interest in human biology or a biology project that you did when you were younger to illustrate your interest in science, and then give examples of how you like to work with others. You should also ensure that you avoid giving reasons relating to money or status; any mention of wanting to be a dentist so that you can earn £200,000 a year is an almost guaranteed way of being rejected!

Your academic interests

It is important for your personal statement to contain information about your academic interests and how they have furthered your desire to study dentistry. This may be related to some topics or practical skills that have been of particular interest to you over the course of your A level studies, or to an interesting article you have read in a newspaper or journal, or to something engaging you heard in a lecture. Whatever it is, it will help to demonstrate your desire to pursue the course, as long as you make it relevant to dentistry.

What have you done to research dentistry?

This is where you can describe your work experience. It is important to demonstrate that you gained something from the work experience, and that it has given you an insight into the profession. You should give an indication of the length of time you spent at each dental practice, what treatments you observed, and the impressions you gained of dentistry. You could comment on what aspects of dentistry attract you, or on what you found interesting or something that you hadn't expected. Beyond this, you should also mention any other work experience you have had in a caring or clinical role and what you learned from it. Although you may not think of these sorts of experiences as being relevant, they can often demonstrate to an admissions tutor good interpersonal skills or commitment and dedication, all of which are relevant to dentistry.

Here is a sample description of a student's work experience that would probably not impress the admissions team.

> 'I spent three days at my local dental practice. I saw some patients having fillings, and a man whose false teeth didn't fit. It was very interesting.'

In contrast, the example below would be much more convincing because it is clear that the student was interested in what was happening.

> 'During my two weeks at the Smith and Smith Dental Clinic, I shadowed two dentists and a hygienist. I watched a range of treatments including fillings, a root canal, extractions and orthodontic treatment. I found particularly interesting the fact that, although both dentists had very different personalities, they both related well to the patients, who seemed to find them very reassuring. A number of things surprised me; in particular, how demanding a dentist's day is.'

It will be far easier to write this section of your personal statement if you spent some time making notes during your work experience. Look back over what you wrote and use your thoughts and experiences as a stimulus for this section. With luck, the selectors may pick up on these experiences at interview and ask you to expand on some of your comments.

In addition to dental-based work experience, admissions tutors now look for evidence of other experience, particularly in a voluntary setting. Any voluntary work is a useful addition to your statement, but voluntary work in a care-based or clinical setting can really help to boost your profile. Opportunities often exist in care homes, children's hospices and hospitals and it is worth trying to contribute regularly over a long period of time rather than carrying it out for just a week or two. This type of experience can help you get an insight into patient care and the communication side of the profession. As with any dental work experience, you should make a note of any key experiences that you have and what they have taught you, as this can then be commented on in your personal statement.

Evidence of developing skills and personal qualities

As a dentist, you will be working with a wide range of professionals and patients throughout your career. To qualify as a dentist, you will study alongside possibly 50 other students in your year, for five years. The person reading your UCAS application has to decide two things: whether you have the right skills and personal qualities to become a successful dentist, and whether you will be able to cope with and contribute to dental school life. To be a successful dentist, you need (among other things!) to:

- be able to survive and enjoy dental school
- have good interpersonal skills and get on with a wide range of people
- be able to work under pressure and cope with stress
- have well-developed manual skills.

How, then, does the person reading your personal statement know whether you have the qualities they are looking for? What you must remember is that the admissions tutor doesn't know you, so you should give lots of evidence of how you have demonstrated and developed these qualities. Some of the things they may be looking for are:

- participation in team events
- involvement in school plays or concerts
- positions of responsibility
- work in the local community
- part-time or holiday jobs
- an ability to get on with people
- participation in activities involving manual dexterity.

What they don't want to hear is how you have demonstrated interpersonal skills by going into town every weekend or how you have improved your manual dexterity by playing PlayStation 3 games!

The selectors will be aware that some schools offer more to their students in the way of activities and responsibilities than others. However, even if there are very few opportunities made available to you through your school, you must still find ways to gain experience and develop your skills. You don't have to have been captain of the rugby team or gone on a three-month expedition to Borneo to be considered, but you do need to be able to demonstrate that you have made efforts to participate in a range of worthwhile activities.

Remember, however, that while evidence of all these skills and extra interests is extremely important, it will not compensate for lower grades, so having a strong academic profile and getting high grades still remain the most important aspects of your application.

Weak and strong personal statements: exemplars

The box on the next page gives an example of a personal statement I have constructed based on experience of reading through what students write. It is made up of a combination of some good ideas, points that need to be expanded on, and things not to say! Overall, as you will probably notice, this would be considered a weak statement and would be unlikely to lead to an offer being made.

DO NOT COPY ANY PARTS OF THESE PERSONAL STATEMENTS!

You should use these examples to give you an idea of structure and the type of content you may want to include, but universities have sophisticated software to detect copied parts of personal statements so do not be tempted! Your personal statement should be personal to you, and, above all else, it should be honest.

Personal statement: Example 1 (character count: 1,523)

I originally wanted to study geography, but realised that there were not many jobs I could go into, so I decided to change my mind and study dentistry. Dentists have to work with people and also in a team and have to have good manual dexterity skills. My motivation to study dentistry is primarily down to money; I have seen how much my dad earns and would like to earn the same. I would ultimately like to pursue a career as a cosmetic dentist as I feel this will allow me to make the most money.

During the Easter holiday, I spent three weeks shadowing a general dental practitioner at my local dental practice. I really enjoyed watching the dentist work and gained a real insight into the skills needed to be a dentist. I also try to keep up to date with the latest developments in dentistry by reading news and journal articles. At the moment I am studying Biology, Chemistry and Psychology at A level. I really enjoy my subjects and feel they will provide me with knowledge and understanding that is particularly appropriate to studying dentistry. I feel that carrying out practical work in biology and chemistry has helped me to develop my manual dexterity skills.

I also have a number of interests outside of school. I like relaxing and enjoy watching TV. I also like going out with my mates at the weekend. I play football in a local league, read science fiction books, play the piano, go to the gym and listen to music. I also have a Saturday job which gives me some extra money to spend when I go out with my mates.

Personal statement: Example 1 raises a number of interesting points.

1. **It is too short.**

   This statement is just over 1,500 characters. The limit is 4,000 characters (including spaces) and you should aim to use as much of this as possible.

   - *It lacks detail and specific examples.*

     The candidate has got the right idea about the structure and addressed the key sections. However, it is very light on actual detail and doesn't really expand on any of the points made or give specific examples. When discussing work experience, go into detail about what you witnessed and what you learned.

When giving details of what you are studying, be specific about topics you have enjoyed. This will give the admissions tutor a much greater insight into who you are and the skills you possess.

- *It is not very personal.*
  This could be about any number of candidates applying to dentistry. Make sure your personal statement has evidence and experiences to show an admissions tutor who you really are.

2. **Never start with a negative.**
   I have seen many personal statements start on a negative point, as is the case here. Any negative points – for example, about things you don't like – do not need to be included. The overall tone should be optimistic and positive.

3. **Don't waste time telling them about dentistry – tell them about you!**
   Statements can often waste time by listing facts about dentistry or what dentists do. Remember that the people reading your statement will know all of this. Use the space instead to illustrate from your own experiences that you possess the qualities and skills that dentists need.

4. **Money should not be your main motivation.**
   Although most dentistry applicants will have thought about how much money they will be making at some point, it is not something that needs to be highlighted in your personal statement. Your reasons for studying dentistry need to run much deeper than this if you are going to get into dental school.

5. **Dentistry is more than cosmetic enhancements.**
   Lots of people fixate on the idea of specialising in cosmetic dentistry. However, dentistry is a far broader discipline and a personal statement should really reflect an understanding of this fact.

6. **Practical work is not the only way of demonstrating manual dexterity.**
   If you are going to use the example of science practicals to demonstrate your manual dexterity, give specific examples of those you have enjoyed or apparatus you have used. You must also try to think of other activities that have helped you demonstrate these skills.

7. **Avoid lists.**
   It can be very easy to simply reduce your work experience and extracurricular activities to a long list. Take time to explain what you gained from each of your placements or interests and how they benefit your application. In addition to this, avoid mentioning mundane interests such as going out with friends and watching TV, because they tell the admissions tutor very little about you.

Although this statement is poor, it would not need much effort to make it a reasonable attempt, as the basic structure is fine. Your first attempt at writing a personal statement will probably be difficult and might not produce great results; however, it is important that you get feedback on your efforts and then redraft the statement as many times as necessary. The best personal statements can take up to 10 drafts to get completely right! Some changes that would be worth making are shown in the following box.

I originally wanted to study geography, but realised that there were not many jobs I could go into, so I decided to change my mind and study dentistry. [*Remove this and try to start on a positive*] Dentists have to work with people and also in a team and have to have good manual dexterity skills. [*They know this! Take the opportunity to show how you have developed and demonstrated these skills*] My motivation to study dentistry is primarily down to money; I have seen how much my dad earns and would like to earn the same. [*Remove the reference to money; instead reflect on other non-financial reasons*] I would ultimately like to pursue a career as a cosmetic dentist and I feel that this will allow me to make the most money. [*Again, remove the reference to money and explain why you are interested in this area of dentistry*]

During the Easter holiday, I spent three weeks shadowing a general dental practitioner at my local dental practice. I really enjoyed watching the dentist work and gained a real insight into the skills needed to be a dentist. [*What exactly did you observe, what did you learn, what interested you?*] I also try to keep up to date with the latest developments in dentistry by reading news and journal articles. [*What have you read about and what topics particularly interest you?*] At the moment I am studying Biology, Chemistry and Psychology at A level. I really enjoy my subjects and feel they will provide me with knowledge and understanding that is particularly appropriate to studying dentistry. [*Be specific about which topics you have enjoyed studying and why they are of interest to you*] I feel that carrying out practical work in biology and chemistry has helped me to develop my manual dexterity skills. [*Which practicals have you enjoyed?*]

I also have a number of interests outside of school. I like relaxing and enjoy watching TV. I also like going out with my mates at the weekend. [*Be imaginative! Nobody is particularly interested in this!*] I play football in a local league, read science fiction books, play the piano, go to the gym and listen to music. I also have a Saturday job which gives me some extra money to spend when I go out with my mates. [*Try to avoid long lists of interests – you will do much better to expand on the really interesting ones; for example, playing piano is the most important here as it demonstrates manual dexterity?*]

Here are two examples of much better personal statements based on those written by two students who both secured entry onto dental courses. Each demonstrates clarity and focus, and what comes through is the enthusiasm that the candidates have for dentistry.

Personal statement: Example 2 (character count: 2,872)

While volunteering in China I was compelled to reflect on the importance of dental care in all our lives. I worked with disabled orphans, many of whom suffered from dental-related pain. It was a humbling experience that made me appreciate the level of dental care I received at home, and how I had taken it for granted. I began research into dentistry and organised several sessions of work experience, giving me a clearer understanding of the everyday demands that dentists face. I am drawn to a career which helps people, allows me to build on my appetite for scientific understanding, and to implement that understanding in a practical way.

I shadowed dentists in general and community dental practices, witnessing simple and restorative treatments; my experiences taught me the importance of good communication skills and the flexibility needed in a surgery. To build on these observations I secured work as a dental receptionist and exercised the skills needed to work with demanding patients. The position required me to work quickly and accurately. These skills were tested by my involvement in the launch of a dental practitioners' accreditation scheme while working as part of the Heart of Birmingham PCT. The aim of the initiative was to encourage implementation of the clinical governance framework to improve levels of customer service in practices.

Volunteering for Dent-Aid enhanced my proficiency as a public speaker and inspired me to work with vulnerable people by carrying out voluntary work for St John Ambulance. As a first-aider, I had the experience of dealing with people with low self-esteem and communication problems; both of these experiences have relevance to becoming a successful dentist and highlighted the importance of empathy when dealing with patients.

At my school, my position as vice house captain was to lead and motivate the house to work together as a team, highlighting both my ability to handle responsibility and leadership skills. Being charity prefect and maths mentor developed my skills in forming relationships, an ability I hope I can transfer to the dental profession. Completing the Duke of Edinburgh's Gold Award furthered my leadership and teamwork skills; I tackled the difficulties we faced with a logical outlook. My determination and persistence are also shown through my achieving 1st and 2nd Dan black belts in karate, and in swimming, in which I have gained gold and honours awards. I achieved 91/95 in my GCSE textiles coursework and my interest in sewing remains as I continue to personalise my wardrobe. My precision and steady hand give me the physical skills needed for a prospective dental student.

I believe that the range of skills I have acquired from my school life and extracurricular activities, as well as my hard-working nature, gives me the potential to flourish as a member of the dental profession.

Personal statement: Example 2, although lacking in some areas, gives a real impression of dedication to pursuing dentistry and demonstrates a very clear and believable explanation of why this student wants to pursue dentistry. They have lots of relevant work experience and really make the most of expanding on what they have learned from it. In addition, this student has picked out the key extracurricular activities and has elaborated on their importance. The small weaknesses are that it doesn't really deal with academic areas of interest and doesn't have too much to say about developing manual dexterity.

Personal statement: Example 3 (character count: 3,874)

I find dentistry to be particularly engaging due to the combination of hands-on patient care and the intellectual creativity that the subject embodies. Furthermore, I feel there is great satisfaction in the pursuit of enhancing and maintaining the oral health of patients in order to develop their confidence and quality of life.

Undertaking work experience at an NHS dental surgery for six weeks altogether has given me direct contact with patients and the oral treatment that they receive. My experience has shown me the importance of informed consent and how essential it is to communicate clearly with patients. At the practice I was able to view a variety of treatments including extractions and root canals. Experiencing these has fuelled my enthusiasm for dentistry and has given me insights into how a dentist deals with problems such as the fragmenting of teeth during extraction. Additionally it revealed the diversity of patients and their problems, proving that it's necessary to be as versatile as possible at all times. Another observation helped me to comprehend the importance of patient information whilst building a diagnosis. In addition I have also given time each week to assist at a dental surgery. This has strengthened my resolve to become a dentist and has made me determined to change people's lives. In the dental surgery I have completed admin duties and have also observed many treatments, which have given me an insight into the complexity of a fully functioning dental team. Moreover, at Birmingham Children's Hospital I undertook work experience for two weeks in various departments including the dental department, accident and emergency and the eye department whilst shadowing doctors, nurses and consultants. This shadowing allowed me to experience a clinical environment and the diverse patient care required at different levels. I learnt the various roles of dentistry in a hospital, for example how important dental care is in treating certain metabolic diseases. Overall, the existence of a multi-disciplinary team came across as essential in a dental surgery in the hospital.

During my A levels I have enjoyed the problem solving involved in studying mathematics, enzymes and immunity in biology, and organic synthesis in chemistry. I have gained various skills while studying, one of those being the ability to look at life from an entirely different perspective due to my understanding of physiology. Additionally I have understood the importance of manual dexterity in a number of experiments I have undertaken, such as monitoring woodlice where the delicate handling of woodlice was required. Also whilst studying I have run an origami club to teach pupils, which lets me practise my manual dexterity skills whilst enjoying myself. Furthermore, as I study I have kept up to date on issues in the dental world, such as all-ceramic crowns, by reading the British Dental Journal, enabling me to advance my interest in dentistry.

I have been a member of St John Ambulance for six months. I've completed first aid courses and volunteered at events which have involved working effectively in a team and building a trusting relationship with patients. Volunteering at Birmingham Children's Hospital for two years has elevated my ability to empathise with patients and adapt to various positions while learning new information.

As a captain at my hockey club I'm responsible for the organisation and cooperation of a team. Similarly, an Envision-funded project presented me with the position of leading and coordinating a team in order to fundraise for Water Aid. Moreover I am a leading member of a youth group in my local area, where I take part in organising debates on world issues. My position as an older member gives me the opportunity to be a role model for the younger ones. Similarly I've counselled pupils at my school as a mentor.

Personal statement: Example 3 has a number of very strong elements. The point of a personal statement is that it should be personal and reflect as much as possible a candidate's individuality; I feel that this statement does this well. The depth of work experience that the candidate has also comes across and helps to show the admissions team that they have really spent time researching the demands of the profession. I certainly get the feeling that this student is genuinely interested in pursuing this career path for the right reasons. On the negative side, the mention of being interested in issues in the dental world feels a little contrived and I would certainly expect this to be developed a little more. I also think that the discussion of academic interests at A level is superficial. However, on the whole a good statement.

Application checklist

- Do you have at least two weeks' work-shadowing experience?
- Do you meet the GCSE entrance requirements for your chosen universities?
- Are you studying the correct combination of A level subjects?
- Are you on target for at least AAA?
- Have you researched the different dental schools and their courses?
- Have you been to university open days?
- Have you completed the UKCAT?
- Does your personal statement demonstrate commitment, research, personal qualities, communication skills and manual dexterity?

What happens next?

- About a week after UCAS receives your application, it will send you a welcome letter and an applicant welcome guide, confirming your personal details and choices. It is vital that you check this information carefully and inform UCAS if there are any inaccuracies. A common mistake is to select the foundation year – the 'pre-dental' year – rather than the start of the course proper, so make sure you haven't done this. Remember, you will be able to access your application at all times through the UCAS Track system using the same personal ID, username and password that you used to apply.

- As soon as UCAS processes your application, your prospective universities can access it, but they will be unable to see the other courses and universities that you have applied to. Once a university has accessed your application, they may contact you to acknowledge receipt of your application; however, not all universities bother doing this, so don't worry if you don't hear from them initially.
- The next stage is to wait to hear from the universities you applied to, once they have considered your application. If you are lucky, you will hear from the dental schools asking you to attend an interview. Some dental schools interview on a first-come, first-served basis, while others wait until all applications are in before deciding whom to interview. It is not uncommon for students to hear nothing until after Christmas, so don't panic if you aren't contacted straight away.
- If you are unlucky, you will receive a notification from UCAS telling you that you have been rejected by one or more of the dental schools. If this happens, don't despair: you may hear better news from another of the schools that you applied to. If you end up with four rejections, you should take the opportunity to carefully reassess whether dentistry is a realistic career ambition for you and whether there were any parts of your application that let you down. If you still feel that dentistry is for you, take the opportunity to strengthen any aspects of your application that were weak, for example undertaking further work experience. Under no circumstances should you give up and decide that it is no longer worth working hard in your academic studies; this will only reduce your chances of making a successful application the following year.
- Note that going through Clearing in August is not an option for entry into dentistry. Places are limited and often oversubscribed, and more offers are made than there are places. There can be the odd exception on a year-to-year basis where a few places are available through Clearing; however, under no circumstances should you bank on any such places becoming available.

6| What makes a successful interview?

Once you've submitted your UCAS application, you must wait to hear from each of the universities you have applied to. If you meet their entry criteria and they like the look of your application, they will probably call you for interview. The universities use interviews to find out first hand whether the picture painted by your application is accurate and to investigate your suitability for their course.

In this section, we will consider both multiple mini and panel types of interview and the specific steps you will need to go through in order to prepare yourself, as well as more general interview pointers. Some of this guidance will be relevant to both types of interview, but differences will be highlighted where necessary.

Multiple mini interviews

In the past, the vast majority of dental interviews have been panel based, where two or more interviewers ask applicants a series of questions. However, in recent years, a significant number of universities have moved towards the system of multiple mini interviews (MMIs), although some still retain the panel style of interview.

The MMI is still designed to judge the suitability of a candidate to study dentistry, and as such will have some similarities with the panel interview; however, the major difference is that applicants participate in a number of small interviews and tasks rather than just sitting in one place answering questions for the whole interview. For example, the MMI at Bristol consists of 10 seven-minute mini interviews, with interviewees rotating from station to station. You are likely to receive instructions at each station explaining what you will be required to do, so ensure that you read them carefully to give you a good idea of what you will be facing.

There are two main reasons for dental schools using this type of interview. Firstly, research has suggested that traditional panel interviews give a poor indication of the likely performance of the interviewee as an undergraduate; the MMI hopes to improve on this. Secondly, one of the major criticisms of the panel interview is that students can be heavily coached on the vast majority of question types and, as a result, do not give an accurate indication of their personality and character attributes at interview. MMIs are therefore specifically designed to test those attributes of the interviewee that are unlikely to be improved by participating in preparation courses. They thereby allow the dental school to build a truer picture of what each candidate is like.

Most universities are relatively tight-lipped about the exact detail of the MMI and give little information to the interviewees. Looking at the details given regarding the MMI at Queen's University Belfast demonstrates this:

'Interviews take the form of short interviews and are designed to test a range of non-cognitive skills such as:

- *maturity and responsibility*
- *interpersonal and communication skills*
- *confidence*
- *self-awareness*
- *empathy*
- *ethical and moral values*
- *awareness of the demands of training as a dental surgeon.'*

Source: www.qub.ac.uk/cm/cms/docs/ admissionprofiledentistry-2011.pdf

Based on this information, it is clear that it is more difficult to thoroughly prepare for an MMI compared with preparing for a panel interview. However, candidates can still take a number of steps to ensure that they are as prepared as possible, even if they will not be fully aware of what to expect. Students should consider the following points in advance of their interview.

- Communication is one of the key skills that will be assessed in the MMI, so you should therefore work on developing your ability to communicate clearly by spending time discussing your application and interest in dentistry with friends, family and an academic adviser or teacher.
- Communicating with different groups of people is a vital skill that dentists need. You should therefore reflect on how you might communicate effectively with different groups of people, for example children, the elderly, or individuals with disabilities.
- Consider your motivation for studying the course. This may be asked directly, but even if it is not, then having a clear idea of your motivation will help to guide your answers to other questions.
- Revisit your personal statement and reflect on key experiences in terms of work experience, leadership, teamwork, motivation, etc.

You should always be prepared to give evidence of how you have demonstrated that you have the skills necessary to be a dentist.

- Practise responding to situations involving ethical dilemmas. An understanding of the standards required of dental professionals can help you to respond appropriately to such situations. These can be found at www.gdc-uk.org/Newsandpublications/Publications/Publications/StandardsforDentalProfessionals[1].pdf.
- Read the invitation to interview letter that the university has sent to you. Often this will give you more details about what to expect on the day and may drop some subtle hints about the interview process.
- Consider and practise the questions that are likely to be asked at a panel interview (see below). Although most of them probably won't come up in the MMI, they will still provide you with opportunities to hone your communication skills and reflect on your experience and motivation. This will help to improve the overall impression you make.

Panel interviews

As discussed above, the traditional panel-style interview is being phased out by a number of dental schools to be replaced by the MMI. Although this type of interview is somewhat easier to prepare for due to the well-known nature of the potential questions, it can be very easy to fall into the trap of memorising pre-rehearsed answers. The questions that are listed below are designed to give you an opportunity to gather your thoughts and reflect on the various aspects of your application rather than devise set answers that you then rehearse and regurgitate in an interview.

Questions for you to reflect on in preparation for your interview

Question: Why did you decide to apply to Shufflefield dental school?

Comment: The panel will be looking for evidence of research, and that your reasons are based on informed judgement rather than just picking a university randomly from a list. Probably the best possible answer would start with 'I came to your open day . . .', because you can then proceed to tell them why you like their university so much, what impressed you about the university and facilities, and how the atmosphere of the place would particularly suit you. If you are/were unable to attend open days, try to arrange a formal or informal visit before you are interviewed so that you can show you are aware of the environment, both academic and physical, and that you like the place. If you know people who are at the dental school or university, so much the better.

You should also know about the course structure; the website and prospectus will give detailed information. Although on the surface all dental courses appear to cover broadly the same subjects, there are big differences between the ways in which courses are delivered and in the opportunities for patient contact, and your interviewers will expect you to know about their specific course.

Answers to avoid are ones such as 'Reputation' (unless you know in detail the areas for which the dental school is highly regarded), 'I don't want to move away from my friends', 'You take a lot of retake students' or 'My dad says it's easy to get a place here'.

Question: Why do you want to be a dentist?

Comment: This is the question that all interviewees expect. Given that the interviewers will be aware that you are expecting the question, they will also expect your answer to be carefully planned. If you look surprised and say something like 'Um . . . well . . . I haven't really thought about why . . .' you can expect to be rejected. Other answers to avoid are those along the lines of 'The money' or 'It's easier than medicine'.

Many students are worried that they will sound insincere when they answer this question. The way to avoid this is to try to bring in reasons that are personal to you: for instance, an incident that sparked your interest (perhaps a visit to your own dentist), or an aspect of your work experience that particularly fascinated you. The important thing is to try to express clearly what interested you instead of generalising your answers. Rather than saying 'Dentistry combines science, working with people and the chance to have control over your career' – which says little about you – tell the interviewers about the way in which your interest progressed.

Here is an example of a good answer.

> 'Although it seemed strange to my friends, I used to enjoy going to the dentist when I was young. This was because my dentist explained things very clearly and patiently, and I was interested in what was happening around me. When I was thinking about my career, I arranged to shadow another dentist, and the more time I spent at the surgery, the more I realised that this would really suit me. It also gave me the chance to find out about what being a dentist is really like. The things about dentistry that I particularly enjoy are . . .'

It is vital that you do not learn this quote and repeat it at your interview. Ensure that your answer is not only personal to you, but also honest.

With luck, the interviewers will pick up on something that you said about work experience and ask you more questions about this. Since 'Why do you want to be a dentist?' is such an obvious question, interviewers often try to find out the information in different ways. Expect questions such as 'When did your interest in dentistry start?' or 'What was it about your work experience that finally convinced you that dentistry was for you?'

Question: I see that you spent two weeks with your dentist. Was there anything that surprised you?

Comment: Variations on this question could include 'Was there anything that particularly interested you?', 'Was there anything you found off-putting?' or simply 'Tell me about your work experience'. What these questions really mean is: 'Are you able to show us that you were interested in what was happening during your work experience?'

Returning to the original question, answering either 'Yes' or 'No' without explanation will not gain you many marks. Similarly, saying 'Yes, I was surprised by the number of patients who seemed very scared' says nothing about your awareness of the dentist's approach to their patients. However, answering: 'Yes, I was surprised by the number of patients who seemed very scared. What struck me, however, was the way in which the dentist dealt with each patient as an individual, sometimes being sympathetic, sometimes explaining things in great detail and sometimes using humour to relax them. For instance . . .' shows that you were interested enough to be aware of more than the most obvious things.

Sentences that start with 'For example . . .' and 'For instance . . .' are particularly important, as they allow you to demonstrate your interest. You should keep a diary of things that you saw during your work experience so that you do not forget and can provide examples. You should then review your diary before interview to refresh your memory.

Question: Can you tell me about something that you have read recently in relation to dentistry?

Comment: If you are interested in making dentistry your career, the selectors will expect you to be interested enough in the subject to want to read about it. Some good sources of information that you may want to make use of are *New Scientist* magazine, the GDC website (www.gdc-uk.org), www.dentistry.co.uk, the BBC news website and broadsheet newspapers. You should get into the habit of checking the news every day to see if there are any dentistry-related stories. Note that the question uses the word 'recently': recent does not mean an article you read two years ago – keep up to date.

Question: During your work experience, you had the chance to discuss dentistry with the practitioner. What do you know about the way NHS dentists are paid?

Comment: You must be aware of the nuts and bolts of running a dental practice; in particular, it is worth understanding the difference between NHS and private work and the way in which the NHS contract system works. You should also have an idea about what a dentist earns and what proportion of it goes back into running the practice. Similar questions might focus on how much dentists are paid for different types of treatment, or how much NHS patients pay for treatment.

Question: Should dental treatment be free on the NHS?

Comment: Although not specifically about dentistry, this type of question can be useful for an admissions tutor to see how you can think on your feet about wider issues. Obviously this type of question needs you to understand what the issues surrounding the NHS are and to have knowledge of what is going on in the world; but more importantly, it needs you to be able to form and express opinions. There is no way you can memorise an answer to this sort of question, as it is not just about recalling facts. If you are struggling to figure out exactly how to respond to such a question, it is worth taking a moment to gather your thoughts before you reply. It is also worth considering both sides of the argument and expressing your reflection on these, as it shows that you have an appreciation of the range of issues involved.

Question: What qualities should a dentist possess?

Comment: Don't simply list the qualities. The interviewer hasn't asked the question because the interviewer is puzzled about what these qualities are; they have asked it to give you a chance to show that you are aware of them, and that you possess them. The best way to answer this is to use phrases such as 'During my work experience at the Smith and Smith Dental Practice, I was able to observe/talk to the dentist, and I became aware that . . .', or 'Communication is very important: for instance, when I was shadowing my dentist, there was a patient who . . .' Always try to relate these general questions to your own experiences.

Question: Do you know what periodontics is?

Comment: There are a range of other questions closely related to this one, aiming to investigate your understanding of some specific areas of dentistry. It doesn't matter whether you are asked about orthodontics, prosthodontics, endodontics or some other area of dentistry, the point is that it gives you an opportunity to talk about your knowledge of the field. This provides another good reason for carrying out careful research into the field of dentistry before applying and for asking questions during work experience. Remember that when you are asked this type of question, the interviewer is not expecting you to have an encyclopaedic knowledge of the area, but is interested in seeing whether you have a solid basic knowledge. It would be worth starting your answer with a basic definition and then, if you have further knowledge or experience of the area, expanding on it. It may also provide another opportunity to discuss a relevant article or current issue that you have seen or to further discuss an experience from a work placement.

Questions about manual dexterity

Question: Dentistry requires a high degree of manual dexterity. How have you developed this skill?

Comment: The question about manual dexterity is very interesting and often ignored by candidates. Manual dexterity means being able to perform intricate tasks with your hands. Dentists have to work in a confined and sensitive area (the mouth) using precision instruments, in situations where accuracy is vital and where there is little margin for error. If you have trouble picking up a coffee cup without knocking it over or if you always press the wrong keys when you work on a computer, dentistry may not be the best career for you. The interviewers will need to be reassured that you have the manual skills to be able to work on other people's teeth. Good examples of tasks that require a high degree of manual dexterity include sewing, embroidery, model-making, touch-typing and playing a musical instrument.

Manual dexterity is a very important factor that should not be overlooked in the selection process. Students, professionals and admissions tutors to whom I've spoken have all indicated that without this quality a prospective candidate might as well not continue with his or her application. If you are not able to give an example of your own manipulative skills, take up a hobby that involves precision work now, before it is too late. Some admissions tutors like interviewees to bring in examples of their handiwork. A particularly good example of this is a student who brought in a denture that she had made during her work experience. This allowed her not only to demonstrate that she possessed the necessary skills but also to talk about the dental technician's role in a dental practice.

Case study 3: Sameera Mukadam

Sameera Mukadam completed her A levels at MPW Birmingham and secured a place at Manchester to study dentistry. Her application was particularly strong due to her extensive work experience and voluntary work, her excellent manual dexterity skills and her interview technique.

'I've always loved studying science and knew I wanted to go into a science-related career from early on in my life. I also didn't want a job that involved sitting behind a desk all day, or in an office answering phones; I wanted something stimulating and exciting that involved meeting new people on a daily basis. After an initial work experience placement at a dental surgery I knew dentistry was what I wanted to do – my experiences there really ignited my passion to follow this vocation.

'I then went on to an ongoing work experience placement at a dental surgery for three months during a summer holiday. It was really eye-opening; I came to realise that dentists have to be prepared for all kinds of situations and are more than just someone who will clean your teeth or take away the pain in your mouth.

'During my A levels, I also carried out ongoing voluntary work at a local hospital every Saturday and Monday morning for 18 months. I was involved in sitting and talking to the patients, making drinks for them and also running errands. Most of the people I helped were old and frail and so it was a real joy to be able to help them.

'Once I had applied to study dentistry, I had two mock interviews to help me prepare and understand the types of questions I was likely to be asked. I also carefully researched the details of the courses I had applied to and tried to keep up to date with the latest dental topics so that I could speak about them if asked in interview. I practised answering questions in the mirror and spent a good deal of time talking to myself!

'My first interview was at Leeds and I really enjoyed it. The panel was very friendly and I really felt I had made a good impression. My Manchester interview was the day after and was the toughest interview I've ever been through! During it, one of the panel asked me about how I would make particular one-molar solutions because I had said on my personal statement that I enjoyed practical chemistry. My advice to prospective dentists is to be totally honest when writing your personal statement, because they are likely to catch you out if you exaggerate any particular points.

'In terms of demonstrating my manual dexterity at interview, I took with me a portfolio of pictures I had taken of the henna hand decorating I had carried out. Over a number of years, I had been involved in fundraisers where I would design patterns for people's hands. I also carried out henna workshops with small children and demonstrated how to do it. My portfolio contained pictures of all of the hands I had decorated and all of the patterns I had designed. I felt that this experience really demonstrated that I had well-developed manual dexterity skills.'

Whatever you do, do not lie about the examples of manual dexterity that you provide. One admissions tutor tells the story of a boy who claimed that he liked icing cakes in his spare time. He brought in photographs of some of the cakes he had iced but it became clear, after very little questioning, that it was his mother who had actually done the work. This did not go down well with the panel, as you can imagine!

Questions to find out what sort of person you are

Question: What interests do you have?

Comment: Don't say 'Watch TV' or 'Go shopping'. Mention something that involves working or communicating with others, for instance sport or music. Use the question to demonstrate that you possess the qualities required in a dentist. However, don't make your answer so insincere that the interviewers realise that you are trying to impress them. Saying 'I relax most effectively when I go to the local dental surgery to shadow the dentist' will not convince them.

Question: How do you cope with stress?

Comment: Dentistry can be a stressful occupation. Dentists have to deal with difficult people, those who are scared and those who react badly when in a dental surgery. Furthermore, there are few 'standard' situations: everyone's mouth and teeth are different, as are their problems, and things can go wrong. In these circumstances, the dentist cannot panic but must remain calm and rational. In addition, the nature of the profession means that the financial aspects of running a business may also be a source of stress. The interviewers want to make a judgement as to whether you will be able to cope with the demands that the course and the job throw up. Once again, be sincere. Reflect on a particularly stressful time in your life and how you have coped through it. Remember, it is always best to use experiences from your own life than to talk generally.

Question: I see that you enjoy reading. What is the most recent book that you have read?

Comment: Although it may sound obvious, if you have written that you enjoy reading on your UCAS application, make sure that you have actually read something recently. Admissions tutors will be able to tell you stories about interviewees who look at them with absolute surprise when they are asked about books, despite reading featuring in the personal statement. Answers such as 'Well . . . I haven't had much time recently, but . . . let me see . . . I read *Elle* last month, and . . . oh yes . . . I had to read *Jane Eyre* for my English GCSE' will not help your chances. The same advice is also true for any other interests you put on your personal statement: if you put it down, you need to be prepared to talk about it!

Other questions to consider

- Why do you want to be a dentist?
- What have you done to investigate dentistry?
- Why does dentistry interest you more than medicine?
- Give me an example of how you cope with stress.
- Why did you apply to this dental school?
- Did you come to our open day?
- During your work experience, did anything surprise you?
- During your work experience, did anything shock you?
- Tell me about preventive dentistry.
- What is orthodontics?
- If you had to organise a campaign to improve dental health, how would you go about it?
- Why do dentists recommend the fluoridation of water supplies?
- What are the arguments against fluoridation of water supplies?
- What are amalgam fillings made of?
- What are white fillings made of?
- There has been a good deal of negative publicity about mercury fillings. Do you think that they are dangerous?
- What is gingivitis?
- How are NHS dentists funded?
- Have you read any articles about dentistry recently?
- What advances can we expect in dental technology/treatment in the future?
- What have you done to demonstrate your commitment to the community?
- What would you contribute to this dental school?
- What are your best/worst qualities?
- What was the last novel that you read? Did you like it?
- What do you do to relax?
- What is your favourite A level subject?
- Do dentists treat children differently from adults?
- What precautions need to be taken with patients who are HIV positive?
- What is an overbite?
- What is the role of the dental nurse/technician?
- How does teamwork apply to the role of a dentist?
- What is the difference between tooth erosion and tooth decay?
- What role does a dentist have in diagnosing other medical problems?
- What are the reasons for the increasing use of composite fillings?

How to succeed in the interview

You should prepare for both types of interview as if you are preparing for an examination. This will involve revisiting your work experience diary so that you can recount details of your time with a dentist and reflect on the key experiences you had and lessons you learned, looking through articles you have saved from the newspaper, the internet and other magazines in relation to dentistry, and considering all the things that you have mentioned in your personal statement. The interviewers are likely to have read your personal statement and may have a copy of it with them, so it is likely that at least one question will pick up on something you mentioned in it. It is therefore vital that you are truthful in your personal statement, as it is very easy to get caught out if you have lied. It is also vital to keep a copy of your personal statement so that you can look over it before your interview; this will enable you to pre-empt some of the points they will raise.

When you are preparing for an interview, try to have a mock interview so that you can get some feedback on your answers. Your school may be able to help you. If not, independent sixth-form colleges usually provide a mock interview service. Friends of your parents may also be able to help. As mentioned previously, do not memorise set answers to questions; this is very easy to spot during an interview and will make you seem insincere. It is much better to have a good idea of roughly what you want to say and then put it across in a natural way. If possible, video your mock interview so that you are aware of the way you come across in such a situation.

At the end of your interview

You may be given the opportunity to ask a question at the end, although this is unlikely in the MMI. Bear in mind that the interviews are carefully timed, and that your attempts to impress the panel with 'clever' questions may do quite the opposite. The golden rule is: only ask a question if you are genuinely interested in the answer (which, of course, is one you were unable to find during your careful reading of the prospectus).

Questions to avoid

- What is the structure of the first year of the course?
- Will I be able to live in a hall of residence?
- When will I first have contact with patients?

As well as being boring questions, the answers to these will be available in the prospectus. If you need to ask these questions, it will be obvious to your interviewers that you have not done any serious research.

Questions you could ask

- Earlier, I couldn't answer the question you asked me on fluoridation of water supplies. What is the answer? (This is something that you genuinely might want to know.)
- How soon will you let me know if I have been successful or not? (This is something you really want to know!)

Remember: if in doubt, don't ask a question. End by saying: 'All of my questions have been answered by the prospectus and the students who showed me around the dental school. Thank you very much for an interesting day.' Smile, shake hands (if appropriate) and say goodbye.

General interview tips

As in any interview, appearance and body language are just as important as the answers you give to the questions you are being asked. The impression that you create can have a big impact. Remember that if the interviewers cannot picture you as a dentist in the future, they are unlikely to offer you a place.

Body language

- Maintain eye contact with the interviewers.
- Direct most of what you are saying to the person who asked you the question, but also occasionally look around at the others on the panel.
- Sit up straight, but adopt a position that you feel comfortable in.
- Don't wave your hands around too much, but don't keep them gripped together to stop them moving either. Fold them across your lap, or rest them on the arms of the chair.

Speech

- Talk slowly and clearly.
- Don't use slang.
- Avoid saying 'Erm . . .', 'You know', 'Sort of' and 'Like'.
- Say 'Hello' at the start of the interview, and thank the interviewer(s) and say 'Goodbye' at the end.

Dress and appearance

- Wear clothes that show you have made an effort for the interview. A suit/jacket and tie (men) or a skirt and blouse (women) are most appropriate and will give the best impression.

- Make sure that you are clean and tidy.
- If appropriate, shave before the interview (but avoid using overpowering aftershave).
- Clean your nails and shoes.
- Wash your hair.
- Avoid (visible) piercings, earrings (men), jeans and trainers.

How you are selected

During the interview, the panel will be assessing you in various categories. Whether or not the interview appears to be structured, the interviewers will be following careful guidelines so that they can compare candidates from different interview sessions.

The scoring system will vary from university to university, but you are likely to be scored in a number of categories, with the dental school setting a minimum mark that you will have to gain if you are to be made an offer. For example, Bristol University gives the following information about the scoring of its MMI interview.

> 'Each MMI station is scored by an assessor on three criteria, giving a total of 30 scores from 10 assessors, and these are collated by the Admissions Tutor to pick the highest-performing candidates. You may have been unsuccessful because you were unable to demonstrate some of the qualities we look for or because your overall score may have been below that of the other interviewees.'
> Source: www.bristol.ac.uk/dental/undergraduates/faq/

If you are below this score but close to it, you may be put on an official or unofficial waiting list. If you are offered a place, you will receive a letter from the dental school telling you what you need to achieve in your A levels: this is called a conditional offer. Post-A level students who have achieved the necessary grades will be given unconditional offers. If you are unlucky, all you will get is a notification from UCAS saying that you have been rejected. If this happens, it is not necessarily the end of the road in dentistry, as you may be able to reapply as a post-A level applicant. What you must do in this situation is contact the universities that you applied to and ask for feedback about why you were unsuccessful. Some universities will be more helpful than others and give relatively detailed feedback, which will give you points to consider. Others will just send you a standard letter with no details about your particular application.

What happens next

When UCAS has received replies from all of your choices, it will send you a statement of offers. You will then have about a month to make up your mind about where you want to go. If you have only one offer, you have two choices. One is to accept the choice and go to that university, happy in the knowledge that you are going to study the course of your dreams; the other is to reject the choice, if you have decided for whatever reason that you don't want to go to that university. If you choose to go down the latter route, you must then apply either the following year or through what is known as UCAS Extra, although it is highly unlikely that places for dentistry will appear on Extra.

If you have more than one offer, you have to accept one as your firm choice, and may accept another as your insurance choice. If the place where you really want to study makes a lower offer than one of your other choices, do not be tempted to choose the lower offer as your insurance choice since you are obliged to go to the dental school that you have put as your firm choice if you achieve the necessary grades. If you narrowly miss the grades required by your firm offer, you may still be accepted on the course. You would have to accept this offer so you would not be able to go to your insurance choice. You can go to your insurance choice only if your firm choice will not accept you. So, if you had put the dental school you really wanted to study at as your insurance choice, in this instance you would not be able to accept a place there.

If you are unsuccessful, there remains the option of completing a first degree and then attempting graduate entry or studying dentistry overseas (see page 89).

Current issues in dentistry

As part of your research into dentistry and during your work experience, you will probably come across news and other articles about a range of current issues related to the profession. While an awareness of what is going on in the world of dentistry may not be of any use in choosing which dental school to apply to, it is absolutely essential when it comes to your preparation for interview, as you will be expected to have a solid understanding of such issues. The aim of this section, therefore, is to give you an idea of some of these issues and provide a starting point for you to do further research. While you are reading and researching, it is important once again to keep a notebook to hand so that you can jot down anything of interest; your notes will then be the perfect starting point for your revision when you receive notice of your first interview.

The nation's oral health

There has been a steady improvement in oral health in the UK. According to the very comprehensive report by the Office for National Statistics, 30% of the adult population had lost all of their natural teeth in 1978, but by 1998 this figure had fallen to 13%. In 1998, adults who still had their own teeth had, on average, 15.8 sound and untreated teeth, compared with 13.0 in 1978. The average number of missing teeth fell from 9.0 in 1978 to 7.2 in 1998. The average number of decayed teeth also fell from 1.9 to 1.0. Reasons for the improvement include:

- fluoridation of water
- fluoride in toothpaste
- developments in dental treatment
- provision of preventive and restorative dental treatment
- increased awareness of dental health.

There has been a significant push by organisations such as the British Dental Health Foundation to raise public awareness of the need for good general oral health. This has been achieved by carrying out educational campaigns such as National Smile Month and providing information to the public regarding issues such as mouth cancer and fluoridation. It is important to recognise the shift from talking about good dental health to talking about good oral health: this represents the fact that it is the health of not just the teeth but of the whole mouth that is important. Promoting the virtues of good oral health in this way continues to have a significant impact on levels of public awareness.

In 2003, a survey into the health of children's teeth revealed that, although it is continuing to improve, there is a big gap between the best and the worst, and some of this is to do with regional differences (www.ons.gov.uk/ons/guide-method/method-quality/specific/health-methodology/dental-health/dental-health-of-children/index.html).

Professor Liz Kay, Scientific Adviser to the BDA (quoted on the BDA's website), said:

> 'While this report does demonstrate a welcome overall improvement in children's dental health, the gulf between those with the best and worst oral health persists. This report shows that a high percentage of our children still suffer unacceptable levels of tooth decay.'

A report in the March 2004 edition of the *British Dental Journal* says that children from Asian backgrounds have healthier teeth. According to the report, over 60% of white children have some tooth erosion, compared with under 50% of children from Asian families. In both groups, boys were more likely to be affected than girls. The report highlights the statistical correlation between high levels of sugar in the diet and levels of tooth erosion. Different dietary habits in the two groups, therefore, might be part of the explanation. One of the major contributing factors towards tooth decay and erosion in children is the consumption of fizzy drinks. According to the BDA, the effect of consuming any fizzy drink increases the chance of tooth erosion in 14-year-olds by 220% (and over 90% of 14-year-olds drink fizzy drinks). Children who drink several fizzy drinks a day increase the chance of damage occurring to their teeth by 500%.

At the other end of the scale, the proportion of over-65s keeping their own teeth is continuing to increase, due to better oral care. According to a study carried out by the BDA, less than a third of over-65s currently have their own teeth; however, this is expected to rise to about 50% within 20 years. The concern is that this rise will put greater pressure on dentists to provide ongoing treatment to a greater number of people.

The National Institute for Health and Clinical Excellence (NICE) has published guidelines on the frequency of dental check-ups. The recommended interval between check-ups has been the same (usually six months) regardless of the patient's age and oral health, but Ralph Davies of the BDA, quoted on the BDA's website, said:

> 'The BDA has always held that the frequency of dental check-ups should be based on the individual patient, not a "one size fits all" system. How often you need an examination should be based on what is best for you as a patient and the clinical judgement of your dentist. NICE has also called for more research to be carried out on this subject and the BDA strongly supports this.'

Mouth cancer

What is mouth cancer?

Mouth cancer is historically thought of as a disease affecting mainly older males; however, over recent years, the incidence in women and children has significantly increased. One of the major issues with mouth cancer is that there is poor public awareness of the disease and its symptoms. Mouth cancer can affect any part of the mouth, including the lips, tongue, cheeks and throat, and has a number of characteristic symptoms, including ulcers that do not heal within three weeks, red and white patches or unusual lumps or swellings in the mouth. A major problem with being able to diagnose and treat mouth cancer is that many people displaying symptoms will ignore them for a long time, thereby delaying effective treatment.

What role do dentists play in relation to mouth cancer?

Early detection of mouth cancer is one of the key factors in successful treatment. This was reinforced by the slogan 'If in doubt, get checked out', used for Mouth Cancer Action Month in 2009. This means that regular screening by dentists plays a vital role in the process of diagnosing and treating those with the disease. This further supports the idea that dentists are responsible not just for treating teeth; they are in fact involved in every aspect of oral health.

What is the incidence of mouth cancer?

According to the BDA, there are around 5,000 new cases of mouth cancer diagnosed annually and roughly 1,800 deaths each year.

Who is at risk?

There are a number of risk factors associated with mouth cancer. However, chewing tobacco or another similar product is the main risk, with excessive alcohol consumption, poor diet and the human papilloma virus (HPV) also being contributing factors. Smoking and drinking to excess is a particular problem because alcohol can aid tobacco absorption in the mouth. This can increase the risk up to thirtyfold.

Tooth whitening regulation

In recent years, there has been a large increase in the number of unregulated tooth whitening treatments administered to the general public. Thousands of people each year have this type of treatment carried out in beauty salons, shopping centres and high streets by individuals with no formal training in tooth whitening. A large increase in the number of complaints made against such companies has led the GDC to call for tooth whitening treatments to be more tightly regulated. In its publication *Considering tooth whitening? What you need to know before committing to treatment* (www.gdc-uk.org/Newsandpublications/Publications/Publications/GDC_Tooth_whitening_leaflet%20(2).pdf), the GDC asserts that any type of whitening treatment constitutes a dental treatment rather than a cosmetic one and as such should be undertaken only by GDC-registered dentists.

Tooth whitening is often carried out to improve the appearance of teeth if staining has occurred due to smoking, drinking tea, coffee and red wine, or just due to age. Common treatments involve using a bleaching gel to make this improvement, but if incorrectly done, this can result in problems such as removing the enamel from teeth and causing gum damage. The GDC and the Department of Health are therefore looking to introduce rules that will allow only dentists or dental-care professionals to carry out such treatments.

The current state of NHS dentistry

What were the 2006 reforms?

The state of NHS dentistry in this country continues to be a hot topic and elicits strong emotions, on the sides of both the professionals and the public. In April 2006, the government carried out sweeping reforms of the system, which were heralded as a new dawn for NHS dentistry and were designed to entice more dentists into the service, thereby improving access to dental care. Under the old system, dentists were paid for each treatment they performed (there were around 400 separate charges), whereas the current system gives dentists a guaranteed income for providing a certain number of courses of NHS treatment to any patient requiring care. The reforms also targeted the pricing system and simplified the structure into three bands, as follows.

- **Band 1 – £17.50:** This charge includes an examination, diagnosis and preventive care. If necessary, this includes X-rays, scale and polish, and planning for further treatment. Urgent and out-of-hours care also costs £17.50.
- **Band 2 – £48.00:** This charge includes all necessary treatment covered by the £17.50 charge, plus additional treatment such as fillings, root canal treatment or extractions.
- **Band 3 – £209.00:** This charge includes all necessary treatment covered by the £17.50 and £48.00 charges, plus more complex procedures such as crowns, dentures or bridges.

Note that in this system, only one dental charge is incurred even if you need to visit more than once to complete a course of dental treatment. If you need more treatment at the same charge level (e.g. an additional filling) within two months of seeing your dentist, this is also free of charge.

Table 5 in Chapter 11 (see page 125) shows a list of different costs, taken from the NHS. You will see in the table that all of the procedures listed fit into one of the three bands. A person pays only once – one charge for each course of treatment. For example, for a check-up, X-ray, teeth polish, a simple filling and a crown, a patient would pay a total of £209 if they all occurred within a two-month period. This pricing structure was designed to try to bring an end to the so-called 'drill and fill' culture and allow dentists to spend more time promoting preventive dentistry.

How were the reforms received?

When the reforms were introduced, many patients welcomed the changes because they felt they would go some way to resolving certain problems associated with accessing NHS dental care, in addition to making the pricing structure clearer. However, the changes did mean that the cost of some basic treatments increased.

Practising dentists were more sceptical of the reforms: a survey of dentists carried out by the BDA in the wake of the changes revealed that 55% of dentists did not think that they allowed them to see more patients. Before the reforms, according to the BDA, 32% of dentists performed 95% of their work on NHS patients, but this fell to 25% of dentists since the reforms. The reforms led to more than 1,000 dentists walking away from NHS work.

What has been the impact of the reforms?

On the whole, the impact of the reforms has been perceived to be negative, with a number of statistics and comments backing this up. Perhaps the most damning statistic that has come to light following the reforms is that, in the two years following their introduction, 1 million fewer patients visited an NHS dentist. In addition to this, according to the BDA, 85% of dentists did not feel that the reforms had improved access. A report from the House of Commons Health Committee also stated that the reforms had not solved the 'fundamental problems'. It has also been implied that some dentists are now less inclined to perform more complex treatments such as crowns and bridges because they receive less money for them.

The BDA said the reforms do not give dentists enough time to do preventive work. This has caused strong feelings among dentists, so much so that in some areas up to three-quarters of dentists are threatening to quit the NHS. According to the BDA, the deal states that dentists must carry out 95% of the courses of treatment which they previously did to get the same money, which dentists say leaves little time for addressing the causes of poor oral health. One of the key issues has been that some dentists have 'used up' the number of courses they have been allocated prior to the end of the year. This ultimately means that they have to turn away any extra patients as they have been given no further funding to treat them.

One dentist I spoke to commented that the NHS does not allow dentists to practise with full clinical freedom and/or reward them for their work, and that until this is sorted out the NHS will remain unattractive to many dentists. As a result, many focus on private practice because this allows greater clinical freedom and more time with patients. In addition, dentists are able to use the best materials and laboratories because any earnings can be reinvested in the business, so, in the end, both patients and dentists are happier.

The 2009 review

In 2009, an independent review of NHS dental services was published that made recommendations about the way forward for dental care in this country. Professor Jimmy Steele, Professor of Oral Health Services Research at Newcastle University, engaged with dental professionals, NHS staff, patients and patient representative groups to compile this review. One of the key changes proposed in the review is that the income of dentists will be determined by three factors – patient list size, quality of care, and the number of courses of treatment rather than just carrying out a set number of courses. In addition to this, the report suggests that patients need to be provided with better information about available NHS dentists and that the three-band pricing structure should be widened to 10 bands. The full report can be found at www.dh.gov.uk/en/Healthcare/Primarycare/Dental/DH_094048.

Following the publication of this report, the government accepted the recommendations 'in principle' and has been piloting them since then. In summer 2011, 62 practices commenced a trial of the new contract with detailed feedback expected in late 2012.

Fluoridation

What is fluoride?

Fluorine is a naturally occurring gas. When fluorine forms a binary compound with another element, this is known as a fluoride. Fluoride ions are found in soil, fresh water and seawater, plants and many foods.

How does fluoride work?

Fluoride is beneficial to both developing and developed teeth, as it decreases the risk of decay. Dental decay is caused by acids produced by the plaque on our teeth, which react with the sugars and other carbohydrates we eat. The acids attack the tooth enamel, which, after repeated attacks, will break down, allowing cavities to form. Fluoride acts by bonding to the tooth enamel, thereby reducing the solubility of the enamel in the acids. Fluoride also inhibits the growth of the bacteria responsible for tooth decay. There is also evidence that it helps repair the very earliest stages of decay by promoting the remineralisation of the tooth enamel. However, fluoride is not a cure-all and the risk of tooth decay can still be increased by other factors such as exposed roots, frequent sugar and carbohydrate consumption, poor oral hygiene and reduced salivary flow.

What is fluoridation?

Fluoride occurs naturally in our water supply at varying levels, usually below 1 part per million (ppm). Fluoridation is the process by which the amount of fluoride is adjusted to the optimum level that protects against tooth decay. Where fluoride is added, the natural level is increased to approximately 1ppm.

What are the benefits of fluoridation?

Initially, the main beneficiaries of fluoridated water supplies were thought to be children under the age of five years. In areas where the concentration of fluoride in water supplies is 1 ppm, rates of decay and tooth loss in children are greatly reduced. High levels of tooth decay in children are generally associated with areas of social deprivation. This is a pattern repeated throughout the EU and the USA. The best dental health regions in the UK are the West Midlands, an area where over two-thirds of the population receive fluoridated water, and south-east England, which is predominantly an affluent area. The worst areas for dental health are those associated with higher levels of social deprivation, such as north-west England. Children living in socially deprived areas with non-fluoridated water supplies can suffer up to six times more tooth decay than those living in more affluent areas or those receiving fluoridated water supplies. For example, in the poorest communities of north-west England, as many as one in three children of pre-school age have had a general anaesthetic for tooth extraction, and in Glasgow tooth extraction is the most common reason for general anaesthesia for children under the age of 10.

Subsequent research has shown that it is not only children who benefit from fluoridated water supplies but people of all ages, as the effect of fluoride on the surface of fully developed teeth is thought to be even more important. Elderly people in particular can benefit from drinking fluoridated water. The decrease in salivary flow with age, combined with reduced manual dexterity, means that it is more difficult to keep your teeth clean as you get older. So older people are more prone to root surface decay, which is difficult to treat. As fluoride strengthens adult tooth enamel, it helps reduce the incidence of this type of decay.

Probably the two most important advantages of fluoridated water supplies, as opposed to any other method of combating tooth decay, are that it is cost-effective and, more importantly, that all members of the community are reached, regardless of income, education or access to dental care.

What are the problems with fluoridation?

The only proven side effect of drinking fluoridated water is dental fluorosis. This is mottling of the teeth caused by a disruption of the enamel formation while the teeth are developing under the gums. It occurs between birth and the age of five years, when the enamel is developing. In mild cases, dental fluorosis is purely a minor cosmetic problem, which is barely visible to either the individual or the observer. It is also thought that mild dental fluorosis may further increase the resistance of the tooth enamel to decay. In moderate to severe cases of dental fluorosis, the colouring of the teeth is very pronounced and irregularities develop on the tooth surface. Whether this is purely a cosmetic problem or whether it adversely affects the function of the teeth is a matter of some debate.

Some research has claimed links between fluorosis and higher instances of bone cancer, osteoarthritis and fractures. However, there have been numerous recent studies by institutions such as the British Medical Research Council concluding that there is no clear evidence that fluoridation of water at the recommended level of 1mg of fluoride to every litre of water causes harm to health, apart from dental fluorosis.

Other concerns expressed about fluoridation are its effect on the environment, particularly on plants. Fluorides have been used in some pesticides and insecticides and their use is now restricted. Other industrial fluorides are one of the main pollutants in lakes, rivers, streams and the atmosphere.

What are the ethical issues involved in fluoridation?

One of the main ethical issues with fluoridation of water supplies involves infringement of personal liberty, as it effectively medicates everyone without an individual having the choice to refuse. We have no choice over our drinking water supply other than through our water company, unless we opt to buy bottled water, the cost of which would be prohibitive for certain sections of the community.

The issue of adding fluoride remains an emotive topic, as demonstrated when the decision was made to fluoridate the water supply of Southampton in 2008. The local health authority decided to introduce fluoridation in an attempt to reduce levels of tooth decay in the city. This plan was carried out in spite of a public consultation that suggested that 72% of 10,000 local people were opposed to the plan. As a result, local residents have mounted a legal challenge, which has the backing of local politicians. Their opposition is based on 'the continuing uncertainties with regard to the long-term health risks associated with fluoridation' and 'the possible adverse environmental effects'.

What is the situation in the UK?

In the UK, around 10% of water supplies are fluoridated. Approximately 6 million people receive optimally fluoridated water, around 3.5 million of whom live in the West Midlands. Other areas with fluoridated supplies are Yorkshire, Trent, Merseyside, Oxford and North-West Thames.

The Water Act 2003 handed the decision of whether to fluoridate water supplies to the strategic health authorities (SHAs) in England and the health boards in Scotland and Wales. The wording states that the decision should be made after 'appropriate public consultation'; a fact that we have seen is not always the case. The Act also means that water suppliers have to comply with the SHA and so have no say as to whether the supply should be fluoridated.

The areas in most need of fluoridated water supplies are those with high tooth decay rates, including Merseyside and other parts of north-west England, Yorkshire, Scotland, Wales and Northern Ireland, plus some socially deprived communities in the south, such as inner London.

Who supports water fluoridation in the UK?

- British Medical Association
- Department of Health
- BDA
- British Association for the Study of Community Dentistry (BASCD)
- British Fluoridation Society (BFS)
- World Health Organization (WHO)
- FDI World Dental Federation

What is the situation in other parts of the world?

According to the BFS, the USA has the most well-developed artificial fluoridation programme in the world, with approximately 171 million people receiving optimally fluoridated water. Other countries with fluoridated supplies are Brazil, Colombia, Malaysia, Canada, Australia, Chile and Korea.

What other products have fluoride added?

Several other methods of increasing fluoride intake have been used, including toothpaste, mouthwash, milk and salt. Salt fluoridation was first introduced in Switzerland in 1955 and is widespread in France, Germany, Austria, Belgium, Spain, the Czech Republic, Slovakia, South America and the Caribbean. This method has the advantage of not requiring a centralised piped water system and gives individuals control over whether they wish to consume it or not.

However, it is not without its problems: dosage must take into account the other sources of fluoride in the area, to ensure that intake is not excessive. The production of fluoridated salt also requires specialist technology. Another consideration is the link between the consumption of sodium and hypertension, which would make this method of fluoride intake unsuitable for some individuals.

Fluoridated milk is also available and has been used (with parental permission) for nearly 40 years in primary schools. Around 42,000 children in the UK, predominantly in the North West, receive fluoridated milk at school, which has a concentration of 0.5mg of fluoride per carton. However, absorption of fluoride from milk is thought to be slower than from water.

Another problem is monitoring and controlling fluoride administered in this manner; it is more difficult than with water because of the number of dairies involved. Fluoridated milk's dosage of fluoride also has to be adjusted, depending on whether the water supply is already naturally fluoridated or not. Additionally, a significant number of people do not drink milk for health or other reasons.

Mercury fillings

What are mercury fillings?

Amalgam fillings, which are the silver-coloured type, are the most common type of metal fillings and have been used for around 150 years. They are made of a combination of mercury (50%), silver (35%), tin (15%), copper and other metals. The major benefit of using amalgam is that it is economical, hard-wearing and long-lasting, and as such is ideal for using on molars.

Are there any risks associated with this type of filling?

There has always been a belief that mercury could not escape from the amalgam, but there is some evidence that mercury vapour does escape. Some countries have banned the use of mercury in fillings, among them Sweden and Austria. Critics of mercury in fillings claim that the vapour can cause gum disease, kidney, liver and lung problems, Alzheimer's disease and multiple sclerosis. However, according to the British Dental Health Foundation, dental amalgam containing mercury is not poisonous when combined with the other metals present. It states that: 'Research into the safety of dental amalgam has been carried out for over 100 years. So far, no reputable controlled studies have found a connection between amalgam fillings and any medical problem.'

What are the alternatives?

The British Society for Mercury Free Dentistry recommends the removal of amalgam fillings and their replacement by composite fillings, but only if precautions are taken to ensure that mercury is not ingested or inhaled. 'White' fillings – made of composite materials or polymers – can be used in place of silver fillings, but they are not as strong and so can often be unsuitable for the back teeth, which are subjected to greater stress than the front teeth. Also being developed is the 'smart filling' – a filling that releases calcium and phosphate ions on contact with acids from the tooth bacteria that cause decay. These ions not only stop the decay, but also help to repair damage.

'Was my treatment necessary?'

Because dentists are paid for the treatment they perform, the more treatment that a patient receives or the more complex the treatment is, the more money the dentist will be able to charge. The question has therefore been raised as to whether dentists provide unnecessary treatment to patients just to make more money. The *Guardian*, in an article entitled 'Do dentists put the bite on patients?', carried out an experiment (albeit a limited one) to test this: a reporter booked examinations at a number of surgeries in London, and the recommendations ranged from one filling and a trip to the hygienist (cost then £32.92) to two fillings and three replacement crowns (£915 then). Even bearing in mind that dentists have to use their professional judgement as to whether treatment is urgently required or could be delayed, the range of recommended treatment in this particular instance is staggering.

The BDA commented: 'Differences in diagnosis are not unusual. It is a matter of judgement and opinion and much will depend on what the patient wants. If you saw lots of GPs you would probably obtain lots of different diagnoses as well.' According to the BDA: 'A dentist's advice about treatment will depend on a number of factors – whether the patient has been seen before, a dentist's understanding of a particular problem the patient might have, the patient's oral hygiene (which might make certain advanced forms of treatment less feasible), the patient's timescale, and so on.'

There have also been suggestions that some NHS dentists can purposely stretch out a course of treatment over more than two months to make more money. Under the current contract, if patients have to return to the dentist within two months to finish a course of treatment or have further treatment, the work is covered by one fee. However, if the treatment goes beyond two months, the dentist would be able to charge again. One Welshman carried out a series of attacks on his dental surgery, including leaving a hoax bomb on its front doorstep, because he thought he had been overcharged by his dentist!

In spite of these concerns and potential issues, it is clear that the great majority of dentists are scrupulous about providing only appropriate treatment in an appropriate timeframe to their patients.

Treatments of the future

Over the past 30 years, the way we have looked after our teeth has improved vastly. We visit the dentist more often, spend more money on dental hygiene products and invest in a wide range of cosmetic dentistry procedures to make our teeth more aesthetically pleasing. As with any other scientific discipline, new treatments and practices are introduced as time goes on and these further improve dental and oral care, and consequently dental health and hygiene. Two recent examples are discussed below.

Coconut and tooth decay

Recent research has suggested that coconut-based products could be used in future dental products to reduce tooth decay. When treated with a specific enzyme, coconut oil inhibited the replication of *Streptococcus mutans*, a bacterium that is a major contributor to tooth decay.

The research, carried out by a group of Irish researchers from the Athlone Institute of Technology, concentrated on the effect of different types of oil in killing the bacteria. It was only the coconut oil that ultimately had any impact. Researchers now wish to see exactly how the oil interacts with the bacteria to cause this effect and how this discovery may be used to influence the next generation of dental products.

Plasma can replace drilling

Currently, dentists use a drill to clean out bacteria from a cavity before inserting a filling; however, a recent article from the BBC suggests that plasma jets could be used in place of drills in the future when carrying out this procedure. Plasma has many natural forms and can be created when energy is added to a gas, using a laser for example. In this case, the bacteria are destroyed by the plasma, but the surrounding tissue remains unaffected. The study found that the low temperatures killed the microbes while preserving the tooth, and also that it was successful even when the bacteria were present as resistant 'biofilms' on the dentine. One of the main benefits to the patient of using this technology is that it is a totally contact-free, pain-free method.

Toothpaste-free toothbrush

Currently under development is a solar-powered electric toothbrush that works without toothpaste. The brush contains a solar panel that transmits electrons to the head of the toothbrush, where they react with acid in the mouth; this creates a reaction that can kill bacteria and break down plaque cells. The research team has tested the toothbrush on bacterial cultures and has found that it causes 'complete destruction of bacterial cells'. The toothbrush will now be trialled.

It is worthwhile trying to keep up to date with advances such as these by reading relevant newspapers, journals and websites. This will enable you to have a good understanding of where the profession is heading and give you the best possible chance of shining at interview.

7| Non-standard applications

Most students who consider pursuing dentistry at university will be classified as 'standard' applicants: these would be UK residents, studying at least two science subjects at A level, and who are applying from school/college or who are retaking immediately after disappointing A level results. However, if you do not fit the profile of a 'standard' applicant but wish to study dentistry, there are other possible entry options that can be pursued.

Those who have not studied science at A level

If you decide that you would like to study dentistry after starting on a combination of A levels that does not fit the subject requirements for entry to dental school, you can apply for the pre-dental course.

The application procedure, the interview and UKCAT requirements are the same as for the five-year course at that particular university.

This course is offered at three faculties of dentistry: Cardiff, Dundee and Manchester (see Table 6 in Chapter 11 for specific details). The course previously offered at Bristol was discontinued in September 2012. The course covers elements of chemistry, biology and physics and lasts one academic year. Following successful completion, you automatically move onto the first year of the undergraduate dental course.

If your pre-dental application is unsuccessful, the best option is to take science A level courses at a sixth-form college. Both state and independent sixth-form colleges offer one-year A level courses that allow you to cover the necessary A levels from scratch. However, covering A level Biology and Chemistry from scratch in one year and getting the required A grades is a very tough challenge and should only be attempted by the most able students. You should discuss your particular circumstances with the staff at a number of colleges to select the course that will prepare you to achieve the A level subjects you need at the grades you require.

Case study 4: Elinor Softley

Elinor is currently in her third year of BDS Dentistry with an integrated foundation year at Manchester University.

'After studying A levels in English Literature, Geography and Psychology, I went on to study psychology and graduated in 2006. I then worked full time for three years in widening participation for Newcastle University and then the University of Sheffield. At Sheffield, I ran a project (the ADOPT scheme) that was designed to encourage students from a variety of backgrounds to consider a career within dentistry. We ran taster days, which incorporated time in clinics, revision sessions, team-building sessions and simulated interviews, alongside an e-learning environment. Through this I worked closely with the dental school, met lots of great staff and got an insight into the careers and, of course, the life of a dental student. I soon found myself wishing I had done dentistry! The hands-on clinical element, and the interaction with a whole host of people on a daily basis really appealed to me. I like fixing things, and I am very much a people person, and I'd like to think I work hard and play hard. The variety of specialisms is huge, and the academic rigour of the course is something that motivates me and challenges me (in a good way!). I didn't want to ever stop learning, and with dentistry you really don't!

'Prior to applying to the course, I undertook a week of work experience at Charles Clifford Dental Hospital, a couple of days shadowing some friends (graduates from Sheffield) in NHS practices around Sheffield and Langold (near Worksop) and a week at a private practice in Gainsborough.

'During these placements, I genuinely felt that dentistry looked like a fantastic career. I was really motivated by the fact that the staff I met along the way genuinely enjoyed their job and highly recommended it to me. I learnt that some patients are open and honest, and will heed any advice you give as a dentist and are genuinely appreciative of the work you do for them. Some are less inclined to undergo the treatments they need, be it for some entrenched fear or lack of motivation to improve their oral health, and you get the impression that the full story is not always being told. Communication skills and approachability are therefore vital in the dentist–patient relationship. No one wants to feel like they are being judged, so getting the balance right and being good at talking to people is a huge element of dentistry alongside the clinical skills required in the field. Work experience also gave me a huge insight into the different specialisms of dentistry (oral surgery, endodontics, periodontics, restorative, maxillofacial surgery) and really revealed just how varied and interesting a career in dentistry can be.

'So far, I absolutely love studying dentistry! At Manchester we get early clinical experience (on each other and on the phantom heads), which is fantastic. I also really enjoy anatomy (we do human dissection) and learning about the physiology of the human body. You get to know your course mates really quickly as the intake is only around 80 undergraduates and the lecturers and academics are approachable and friendly. As long as you attend all your classes, and put the hours of private study in, then it is not too big a mountain to climb.

'My main tips for prospective dental students are to be yourself at interview and do lots of work experience to see if this really is the path for you. Don't do it for your parents, or "for the money" – do it because you genuinely want to bring something to the profession. You're a long time dead, as the saying goes, and your working life will take up an enormous chunk of your existence on this planet, so choose your path wisely and do what makes you happy.'

Overseas students

The competition for the few places available to overseas students is fierce and you would be wise to discuss your application informally with the dental school before submitting your UCAS application. Many dental schools give preference to students who do not have adequate provision for training in their own countries. You should contact the dental schools individually for advice.

According to the UCAS entrance statistics, students applying from outside the UK are much less successful than their UK counterparts in getting offers to study dentistry. For entry in 2011, around 93 overseas students (EU and non-EU) gained a place to study at British universities, out of 473 applications. This represents a 20% chance of success compared with a 43% chance for UK students who applied in the same year. Further breakdown of these figures shows that around 28% of non-UK/EU students gain places, and about 6% of EU students are successful. There are a number of reasons for this and these are discussed below.

Qualifications

Many overseas students are applying with qualifications that are not equivalent to A levels or other UK qualifications. These students cannot be considered unless they have done a course that leads to qualifications recognised as being equivalent to A levels, such as International Baccalaureate (IB) or the Irish Leaving Certificate. The dental schools' websites will quote entrance requirements in terms of A levels, IB, Scottish Highers, the Irish Leaving Certificate and other equivalent qualifications. If you are studying for other qualifications, you will need to contact the dental schools directly to ask their advice. The UCAS website also has a link to the UK government's education qualifications website, where you can check whether your examinations are suitable.

If not, you will need to think about following a one-year A level pro-gramme (studying Biology, Chemistry and another subject) and applying while studying. Students will also need to demonstrate proficiency in English and in most cases will be asked to have an IELTS (International English Language Testing System) score of at least 7.0.

The application form

Students who are studying outside the UK are often at a disadvantage because they may not have access to advisers at their schools who are familiar with the requirements of a successful UCAS application. The two areas that tend to be weakest are the personal statement and the reference.

Students who are unfamiliar with UCAS applications often write unsuit-able personal statements that concentrate too much on non-essential information (prizes, awards, responsibilities) and not enough on matters relevant to dentistry. It is important to explain why you wish to study dentistry in the UK rather than in your home country. Detailed advice on the personal statement can be found in Chapter 5 of this book. Simi-larly, your referee needs to be familiar with what the dental schools require in the reference. The UCAS website contains a section with information for referees: you should ensure that your chosen referee is familiar with this.

Work experience

Dental schools almost always require applicants to have gained some relevant work experience, and often to have done some voluntary work as well. Work experience tells the selectors that the candidates are serious about becoming dentists and that they are familiar with what the profession demands. Voluntary work demonstrates that the applicant has the caring nature necessary to work with patients. Gaining work experience can be difficult, but you should make every effort to do so. If it is impossible for you to gain dental work experience, you might try to substitute it with hospital work or by attending relevant lectures. It is important that the reference explains why there is no mention of work experience in the application, and what you did to try to get that experience.

In addition to trying for work experience, there are short courses run in hospitals by dentists giving an insight into the profession. This is particularly useful for those who are not convinced that dentistry is the right profession for them, and also for those who have made up their minds but want greater insight and a good talking point for interview. Visit www.mdexperience.co.uk for further information on these short seminars.

Interviews

Most dental schools require students to attend interviews. This is often difficult to arrange for students who are not based in the UK. It is worth contacting the schools before you apply to see whether they are likely to require you to travel to the UK to be interviewed.

Quotas

While there is no restriction on places for EU students (who will be considered alongside UK applicants), the UK government imposes quotas for non-UK/EU students. For example, Sheffield accepted only four non-EU international students for entry in 2011. In general, students from countries that do not have adequate training programmes for dentistry are likely to have an advantage. If you are serious about studying dentistry in the UK, then do not be put off by the statistics. It is worth bearing in mind that while almost all of the UK applicants will be suitably qualified to study dentistry and will be aware of the entrance requirements (academic and other), a high proportion of overseas applicants will be rejected simply because they have not researched the requirements properly. So, careful preparation will give you a good chance of being considered. In 2011, around 81 non-EU overseas applicants were successful, and many go on to have a long and fruitful career, often staying in the UK.

Mature students

Every year, there are a number of entrants to dentistry who are mature students. In 2011, there were around 277 students aged 22 or over who gained entry onto a dentistry course. In general there are three types of mature student:

1.   those who have always wanted to study dentistry but who failed to get into dental school when they applied from school in the normal way

2. those that have studied a science-related degree and at some point decided that they wish to study dentistry

3. those that came to the idea later on in life, often having embarked on a totally unrelated degree or career.

The first two types of applicant will usually have completed a degree in an associated discipline, such as a science or healthcare-related subject, and usually will have obtained a minimum classification of 2.i. This may be because they did not get into a dental school when they applied as an A level student, or simply because they wanted to pursue a science degree without ever really considering dentistry at the time. Applicants who want to consider this route will have a greater chance of success if they have pursued an appropriate biomedical or healthcare-related first degree, such as:

- anatomy
- biomedical sciences
- biochemistry
- human biology
- medical science
- physiology.

This is intended as a guide only, and the suitability of any degree course should be checked directly with the university.

This type of applicant would then apply to one of the four-year graduate-entry courses following completion of their first degree. This type of course is offered by Aberdeen, Central Lancashire (UCLan), King's and Liverpool. These courses offer exemption from the first year of the course, so entry is into year two. Students who opt for this path can face an uphill struggle to make a successful application and so would need to have an excellent profile that demonstrates ongoing commitment to dentistry to maximise their chances of being accepted. Table 7 in Chapter 11 gives details of these courses.

The second category of mature student is of equal interest to the dental school selectors and interviewers. Applications from people who have achieved success in other, non-science-related careers and who can bring a breadth of experience to the dental school and to the profession are welcomed. The main difficulty facing those who come late to the idea of studying dentistry is that they rarely have scientific backgrounds. There are two possible pathways that can be considered if you are in this position. Firstly, it would be possible to study science A levels and apply for a five-year course. Independent sixth-form colleges would be best placed to provide this pathway. Alternatively, it would be possible to apply to one of the six-year dental courses that incorporate a pre-dental year. These courses are offered by Cardiff, Dundee and Manchester and are open to those who have achieved grades AAA at A level but have studied only a maximum of one science A level.

Case study 5: Joanne Lamb

Joanne Lamb is a medical graduate from the University of Sheffield and is currently studying dentistry there as part of her training for maxillofacial and oral surgery.

'I find dentistry far more practical than medicine, with much earlier patient contact and responsibility for patients in terms of treatment planning, booking appointments, lab work and general timekeeping and organisational skills. It is important to realise that dentistry is not as narrow a subject as some people might think; there are a wide range of specialties and also lots of general medicine in the course.

'My advice to prospective dentists would be to use your general life experiences to your advantage on your personal statement. Do not just list your hobbies – talk about what they teach you. Everything can be turned into something positive – a student on an open day the other day asked me whether art A level was relevant as a fourth subject. I told him to definitely mention it as dentistry is very arty – quite a lot of "sculpture" is involved when trying to rebuild teeth. Also, make sure you don't just concentrate on academic achievements in your statement or interview – everyone will have the grades, so what makes you different? I would also suggest trying to get some work experience on top of clinical experience – maybe working in a dental tech lab, as this can provide valuable extra background.'

Studying abroad

One option for those who have been unsuccessful with their applications is to study dentistry at one of a number of dental schools abroad. These are five- and six-year courses that are taught in English and are recognised by the UK's GDC. The most well known of these universities are Charles University in the Czech Republic and Comenius University in Bratislava, capital of Slovakia, although there are many other courses available. There is no central body like UCAS to apply through for these schools, so applications are completed individually for each dental school. The admissions process can differ for each university, but there may be the requirement to sit an entrance exam and/or attend an interview.

It is advised that students who are interested in studying abroad start their research up to 18 months in advance. This will allow enough time to thoroughly complete any application forms, sit any required tests or entrance exams (including language tests), obtain a visa (if required) and find funding. There are different guidelines to follow depending on where you wish to study and you will also need to research exactly what it is that you need to do. For example, if you wish to pursue a course within the EU and you are an EU national, you have a right to study in any other EU country. You also have the right to be charged the same level of fees that a home student in that country would pay. This means that the process is relatively straightforward, and there is no requirement to apply for a visa.

If you wish to study outside the EU, however, there may be a requirement to apply for a student visa. You may also find that you have to pay different fees compared with students who originate from the country. It is vital that you speak with the embassy or consulate of the country you wish to study in to check the steps that need to be followed.

There are some companies based in the UK that aim to help you gain entry to one of a number of these universities; however, it is best to approach the university directly to discuss entry as this is often a more straightforward and less expensive option. Applicants who are offered a place to study dentistry in Europe are not obliged to accept their place if they later choose to study in the UK. It is advisable for any committed prospective dentist who is applying for a UK dental school to have a back-up option to study dentistry in Europe, in the event that their application in the UK is unsuccessful.

The UK Council for International Student Affairs (UKCISA) website (www.ukcisa.org.uk) is full of useful information and is a good place to start your research.

When considering study abroad, you should take time to investigate whether the course you will be studying is recognised by the GDC and will lead to full registration. Dentists who have a degree from a country in the European Economic Area (EEA) are likely to be able to register with the GDC on the basis of that qualification. However, you should still make sure that you check with the GDC the standing of any course within the EEA that you are considering studying, particularly if you are considering Bulgaria or Romania.

If you study outside the EEA and your qualification is not recognised for full registration with the GDC, upon graduation you will need to take a test called the Overseas Registration Examination (ORE). This will test knowledge and clinical skills based on the curriculum of UK dental schools. If you pass, you are then eligible to apply for full registration.

Case study 6: Samera Altaf

'I am currently studying dentistry at UMF University in Cluj-Napoca, Romania, and am about to go into my third year. I chose to study dentistry as I have always enjoyed carrying out practical work and using my hands. I also feel that dentistry is a real art and this has always appealed to me. I have also been inspired by observing my brother's career as a dentist and seeing the enjoyment that he always gets out of it. During my A levels, I carried out a number of work experience placements that also gave me a real feel for what it would be like to be a dentist; this just served to further my desire to pursue this course.

'Deciding to study abroad was a daunting prospect initially. Despite having two brothers already established in Romania on their respective courses, I had reservations about how I would acclimatise – not only to university life but also to a whole new country. I was particularly nervous about the language barrier, studying with a different course structure and the cultural and social differences. However, having been there now for two years, I feel the positives of studying abroad far outweigh the negatives: I have met people from all walks of life, learned a new language and found out about a whole new culture. On a personal note, I have acquired more self-assurance and independence since I started studying here. The only real negative is that I am far from family and friends and I find I often miss them.

'So far, the course has been really hard work and there has been a lot to learn and take in. However, I am finding it really enjoyable, particularly my study of subjects such as anatomy and dental morphology. I also enjoy the labs, as they include working with teeth and dental materials, which is very interesting.'

Case study 7: Manav Gupta

Manav is currently studying at Charles University in Prague and has just started his second year.

'I have always wanted to be a dentist as it has everything that I want in a career. I have always enjoyed practical subjects and really look forward to working as part of a team to help people maintain and improve their oral health. Although I have always had this interest in dentistry, I made sure that I carried out extensive work experience so that I was prepared for what would lie ahead. I saw NHS and private practices as well as shadowing in the maxillofacial department of my local hospital. I also particularly enjoyed shadowing a dentist in India. On the whole, I was amazed by the importance of manual dexterity skills; while I knew that there would be a massive practical element, I had somewhat underestimated how important these skills were for a dentist to be successful.

'So far, I am really enjoying learning about dentistry and love the practical classes. The other subjects such as histology and anatomy are not so interesting, but it is important to see how they fit into the bigger picture.

'Before considering studying abroad, students should understand that the courses are not easy! This option does not provide a route that anybody can follow successfully – you need to be academically very able and highly motivated. Even with my A level grades of A*AA, I have still struggled to keep on top of my workload. The pass marks for tests and assignments can also be very high and the intensity of the course can leave lots of students stunned!

'One of the things that I was surprised by was the level of importance placed on memorising factual detail. This was a bit of a shock as my A levels were a lot more about applying knowledge rather than just regurgitating it. As a result, I initially found it difficult to relate to and enjoy, as all I was doing was memorising pages from a book.'

Students with disabilities and special educational needs

Students with disabilities and special educational needs are welcome to apply to study dentistry. The vast majority of universities will have an equality and diversity adviser or team (or equivalent) that is employed to provide guidance and support to students with specific needs.

It is absolutely vital that any specific learning difficulty or disability is disclosed in the appropriate section of your UCAS application. It is crucial that no details are hidden from the university at this point. If the university knows about your needs from the start, they will be better placed to provide the appropriate support from the beginning of your course. It is also important to remember that your application will not be discriminated against based on the information you provide in it. The University of Sheffield nicely summarises this on its website by saying:

'Your application is considered on an individual basis and no pre-sumptions are made about a disability and how it may affect you in relation to your chosen course. Your academic merit, potential and abilities will be considered first and foremost.'

All universities will have similar policies in place to ensure that there is no discrimination throughout the process.

It must be remembered, however, that dentistry makes very specific physical demands on individuals. As a result, any physical disability that may interfere with the ability to meet these demands may make dentistry an unsuitable course. The GDC recommends that a student should only be accepted onto a course if he or she is able to carry out all of the tasks normally done by dentists. They also require applicants to satisfy the 'fitness to practise' criteria. If you are unsure about how your disability will affect you in these areas, then it is worth contacting the universities so that you can be assessed individually.

It is also worth contacting the team at each university where you wish to study in advance of applying to discuss the facilities and mechanisms they would be able to put in place to support you during your studies. This is a vital task and so should form part of your research and fact-finding about a particular university.

8 | What do I do on results day?

You will probably have been worrying about results day for a number of weeks by the time it eventually rolls around. Although it can be a very emotional day for some, it is important to be thoroughly prepared to deal with whatever situation may arise on the day.

Your A level results will usually arrive at your school on the third Thursday in August, with the dental schools receiving them a few days earlier. Scottish Higher results are traditionally released a week earlier than A level results. It is vital that you are present in person on the day so that you can collect your results; don't wait for your school to post them, and try to avoid getting them by phone or email as this can sometimes lead to you being given incorrect information. Collecting your results at school will put you in the best position to act as quickly as possible if you haven't managed to secure your place. Prior to results day, check what time your school opens and what time results are available; the sooner you get to your college and pick them up, the sooner you could be on the phone to university admissions teams. In addition to this, you will be able to find out whether you have been accepted or rejected from your chosen universities prior to going into your school or college by logging on to UCAS Track, so have your login details to hand.

If you received a conditional offer and your grades equal or exceed that offer, congratulations! You can relax and wait for your chosen dental school to contact you with details of accommodation and other arrangements.

What to do if you hold no offer

There are a number of students who will approach results day without having received an offer from a dental school. In the past, if you found yourself in this position and secured excellent grades in your A levels, it may have been possible to find a place through Clearing. Unfortunately, it is now virtually impossible for a student to secure a place on a dentistry course in this way, even if they hold outstanding grades. This situation is unlikely to change in coming years. Ultimately, though, Clearing may be of use to secure a place on an alternative course.

If you hold three A/A* grades but were rejected when you applied through UCAS (i.e. you did not get an offer), you need to let the dental schools know that you are out there, and discuss options for how you may secure a place in the future. The best way to do this is by phone or email, as these are the quickest ways of contacting the dental schools directly. It is always best to try to establish a good working relationship with admissions tutors and admissions teams at the universities you are interested in, as they will be more likely to give you advice and help you in the future.

In this situation, the main option you have is to reapply through UCAS in the next admissions cycle. Although you will already have the grades for entry in this situation, it is important to understand that there are a number of other elements of your application that you'll need to work on to maximise your chances of securing a place. Things to consider are listed below.

- Your personal statement: revisit it and cast a critical eye over it. This is also an opportunity to add any work placements or other positive experiences that you have had since your last application.
- Your UKCAT score: you will need to resit your UKCAT for each admissions cycle. This will give you a chance to complete further practice questions and learn from your experience of sitting it first time around. It may also be a good idea to attend one of the UKCAT preparation courses that are available.
- Your work experience: any opportunity to add further work experience to your profile will always be a good idea. Whether it is dentistry-related or just general voluntary work, it will have a positive impact.
- Evidence of manual dexterity: if you were called to interview, would you have evidence of your high degree of manual dexterity? If not, the gap between results and applying again is an ideal time to develop an interest that could support this.

Is the Adjustment facility on the UCAS website of any use to me?

In effect, the UCAS Adjustment option is designed to be a 'trading up' system for applicants who pass their exams with better results than expected. However, you can only enter Adjustment if your results have met and exceeded the conditions of your conditional firm choice. A student must have held a conditional firm choice on their application to be eligible, and so if you have had no offers it is not something you can use.

What to do if you hold an offer but miss the grades

If you have only narrowly missed the required grades, it is important that you contact the dental admissions team as soon as possible. As mentioned previously, you will probably know what their decision is at this point, thanks to the UCAS website. If you have been rejected, it is vital that you keep a level head and do not panic; you must stay calm throughout. If you have not been rejected outright or are unsure of their decision, you must contact the admissions team by telephone – so ensure that in the run-up to results day you have gathered together the contact numbers of the universities you have accepted as your firm and insurance choices.

In some cases, dental schools will allow applicants who hold a conditional offer to slip a grade (particularly if they came across well at the interview stage) rather than offering the place to somebody else. However, be warned – this is a rare occurrence and most of the time dropping a grade will result in outright rejection.

When speaking to the universities, they are likely to give you a simple yes or no answer or tell you that you are still being considered. It is unlikely that crying, begging or pleading your case to the person on the phone will make any difference to the overall decision. If they tell you that you have been rejected, there are some questions you should ask.

- Would they consider your application if you applied next year (i.e. do they accept resit students)?
- What would the likely grade requirements be?
- Would they interview you again?

If they have given you a positive response about reapplying, seek to get it confirmed in writing, as this will give you hard evidence of their intention to consider your application again. It is probably easiest for them to confirm this by email, so you will first need to send them an email to enquire. If you are told by the universities you held offers with that they will not consider your application in the next cycle, you should call other dental schools to see if they would consider you. Unfortunately, the number of dental schools that will consider applications from retake students who have not held a conditional firm offer with them is becoming more limited every year (see Table 2 in Chapter 11, page 120).

If you have had a positive response from one or more dental schools about reapplying, you would then need to consider retaking your A levels and applying again later in the year (see below). The alternative is to use the Clearing system to obtain a place on a degree course related to dentistry and then apply to the dental course after you graduate and hope to be offered a place. Remember: as previously mentioned, entry onto dentistry courses through Clearing is no longer an option.

Retaking A levels

If you narrowly miss the required grades in your A levels after two years of study, you may wish to take the opportunity to retake any subject in which you underperformed to try to boost your grade. Remember that it is extremely difficult to make a successful application as a retake student, so improving your grades may not be enough to get you into dentistry. However, if you held offers with dental schools in the previous year and only narrowly missed your grades, you are more likely to be considered again the following year.

In terms of what you should retake, it is best to take advice from the college that is preparing you for the retake. In some cases, you might be close enough to the grade boundary to risk retaking just one unit; but bear in mind that the more units that you retake, the fewer extra marks you have to achieve in each to reach the A grade boundary. It is also worth remembering that A2 units are harder than AS units, so you are more likely to be able to gain the extra marks that you need by retaking an AS unit or two than by relying on the A2 units alone.

It is worth taking note that from January 2014, AS and A level units can no longer be taken in January. Most retake students will need to resit exams in the summer exam session. If you are retaking course-work units you need to check when this can be done with the exam board.

Numerous state and independent sixth-form colleges provide specialist advice and teaching for students considering A level retakes. Interviews to discuss this are free and carry no obligation to enrol on a course, so it is worth taking the time to talk to staff before you embark on A level retakes.

Reapplying to dental school

Most dental schools do not consider retake candidates (see Table 2 in Chapter 11, page 120), so the whole business of applying again needs careful thought and research, hard work and a bit of luck.

When reapplying, the choice of dental schools open to you will be narrower than the first time round. Most do not consider retake students at all; others will only consider you if there are extenuating circumstances that affected your academic performance; while some will only consider you if you previously applied to study with them and were made an offer. It is vital that you check the advice given by each dental school before you think about applying to them, as their position on retake students is always changing.

If you feel that there are extenuating circumstances that have prevented you from reaching your target grades, you must try to get evidence to support this. For example, if you have had a medical condition that has affected your performance, a letter from your doctor will be sufficient. Some examples of acceptable reasons for underachieving are:

- your own illness
- the death or serious illness of a very close relative.

The following are examples of excuses that would not be regarded by admissions tutors as extenuating circumstances.

- 'I had so many exams to revise for that I didn't have time to do everything.'
- 'I have three young brothers and the noise they make stops me from revising.'
- 'I went skiing at Easter, and was unable to revise properly because it was too cold in the evenings for me to work.'
- 'I lost all of my notes a week before the exam and so couldn't revise.'
- 'We moved house a month before the exams, which disrupted my revision schedule.'

These are just guidelines, and the only safe method of finding out whether a dental school will consider your application is to call or write and ask. It is often worth writing an email or letter so that you have firm details of what has been discussed to refer back to at a later point if necessary. An example is provided on page 100, although a telephone discussion could also take this form. Don't follow it word for word, and do take the time to write to several dental schools before you make your final choice. The format of your email should be:

- an opening paragraph
- your exam results: set them out clearly and with no omissions
- any extenuating circumstances (a brief statement)
- your retake plan, including the timescale
- a request for help and advice
- a closing paragraph.

Make sure that your letter is brief, clear and well presented. If you have had any previous contact with the admissions staff you will be able to write 'Dear Dr Smith' and 'Yours sincerely'. Even if you go to this trouble, the pressure on dental schools in the autumn is such that you may receive no more than a standard reply to the effect that, if you apply, your application will be considered. Apart from the care needed in making the choice of dental school, the rest of the application procedure is as described in the first part of this guide.

Remember that if you are reapplying to universities that use the UKCAT, then you will also have to resit the test, regardless of how you did in the previous year. Unlike your A level modules, it is not your best scores that will count, rather your most recent ones.

Dear Miss Nash

Last year's UCAS No. 08-123456-7

I am currently in the process of completing my UCAS application and am particularly interested in applying to Shufflefield to study dentistry. I applied to you last year and received an offer of AAB but missed the grades/was rejected after interview/was rejected without an interview. However, I am very impressed by the university and the structure of the course and as such would like to apply again. I have just received my A level results, which were Biology A, Chemistry B, Psychology B. I also have a grade B in AS English Literature.

During my final year of A levels, I had significant health problems that prevented me from achieving the grades I am capable of. I am now embarking on a 16-week course in each of my subjects so that I can improve my grades. Now that I am back to full health, I have no doubt that I can achieve A grades in each subject.

Could you please advise me as to whether you would consider my application, given the circumstances I have outlined above. I am very keen not to waste a slot on my UCAS application (or your time) by applying to you if you will reject me purely because I am retaking.

I am very keen to come to Shufflefield, and would be extremely grateful for any advice that you can give me.

Yours sincerely

Diana Littlewood (Miss)

9 | Fees and funding

Whether undertaking an undergraduate or postgraduate course, the cost of studying is considerable. This has been exacerbated in recent years by rises in living costs and the large increases in university tuition fees following the Browne review. A study of 2,800 students (www.bbc.co.uk/news/education-14488312) estimated that average debt upon graduation could reach £53,000 per student; however, this was based on an average course length of 3.4 years, rather than the 5 years it takes to complete a dentistry degree. If we take into account the course length, then an English student at an English dental school outside London could leave university with a minimum debt of £72,500 if the full amount of student loan is received and there is no financial support from other sources. Bear in mind, however, that this overall cost will fluctuate depending on a number of factors. Some of these are listed below.

- Geographical location: obviously studying in London is going to be more expensive than studying in Birmingham.
- Area of permanent residence: there are differences in fees payable and help available depending on where you are from.
- Parental help: contributions from parents may significantly help meet the cost of living.
- Eligibility for grants: means-tested grants can help to reduce the overall cost of living.
- Availability of scholarships: does the university offer scholarships for exceptional students?
- Finding a job: although it has the potential to interfere with your studies, working during your time at university will help to reduce the overall burden of debt.

When considering levels of student debt, it is easy to become disheartened and think that university study is not for you. I commonly hear students saying that they can't afford to go to university as they don't have the money to pay for it. What all students must remember is that tuition fees do not have to be paid up front; in fact, most students receive student loans to cover this cost. In addition, the loans do not start to be paid back until you are earning over a certain amount. The full details of this will be discussed later in the chapter.

Regardless of how much debt you incur, or how you fund your way through university, hopefully these figures will help you to realise that undertaking a course such as dentistry should only be done after seriously considering the overall cost and carefully examining your ability to be fully committed to your study for the full five years.

To find out what the fees are and what funding is available for dentistry courses, you should explore each of the universities' websites and/or talk to their financial departments, because fees and funding procedures vary from university to university. You must also ensure that you plan your finances carefully in terms of tuition fees, living costs, and books and other necessary equipment. Needless to say, living costs in big cities such as London will be much higher than in other parts of the country.

Fees

UK

Students who are UK nationals pay lower tuition fees than non-EU international students. From September 2012, universities can charge up to the maximum tuition fees of £9,000 per year, although these may continue to rise in the future.

There are a number of differences between the systems in England, Scotland, Wales and Northern Ireland, which can result in massive differences between the fees that are ultimately paid by students. For September 2012, the rules are as follows, although they may be subject to change in the future.

- English students are liable for the full fees being charged regardless of where they study within the UK.
- Students living in Scotland who wish to study full time at a Scottish university are not required to pay tuition fees as long as eligibility criteria are met. Scottish students who wish to study at a university in England, Wales or Northern Ireland are required to pay fees of up to £9,000 per academic year.
- For students residing in Wales, a non-repayable, non-means-tested grant from the Welsh government of £5,535 per academic year will be available. This therefore means that Welsh students will effectively pay tuition fees of up to £3,465 per year, regardless of where they study in the UK.
- Students living in Northern Ireland who wish to study in Northern Ireland will pay £3,465 per academic year. Northern Irish students who wish to study elsewhere in the UK are required to pay up to £9,000 per academic year.

EU students

EU students, not including those living in the UK, can expect to pay different levels of fees depending on where they study in the UK. For September 2012, the rules are as follows.

- EU students studying in England will pay up to £9,000 per year, depending on the course.
- In Scotland, these students are not required to pay tuition fees as long as they meet eligibility criteria.
- In Wales, EU students can receive a grant of £5,535, meaning that they effectively pay up to £3,465 per year.
- In Northern Ireland, EU students pay £3,465 per academic year.

Non-EU international students

For international students from outside the UK and EU, the costs of studying in the UK are significantly greater and can often be prohibitive. For example, at the University of Manchester the tuition fees for students starting in the academic year 2012–13 are £15,400 for the first year and £28,200 per annum for years two to five. The University of Glasgow charges £28,500 per annum. While there is some variation in cost between universities, these fees are broadly representative of the whole of the UK.

Financial help

There are a number of sources of financial help that are potentially available for full-time students from both the UK and EU to help cover the cost of university study. The main ones are student loans, grants and bursaries, which are all allocated according to individual and family circumstances. It is important to apply as soon as possible through the Student Finance online service in order to prevent delay in receiving this assistance. There are different Student Finance sites to use depending on which country you are a permanent resident of. These sites contain detailed information on the help that is available and how to apply for it:

- **England:** Student Finance England – www.studentfinanceengland. co.uk
- **Scotland:** Student Awards Agency for Scotland (SAAS) – www. saas.gov.uk
- **Wales:** Student Finance Wales – www.studentfinancewales.co.uk
- **Northern Ireland:** Student Finance Northern Ireland – www.student financeni.co.uk

For the most recent figures, please check the relevant Student Finance websites regularly.

Student loans

The most common way for students to finance their studies is by taking out a student loan. If you are an eligible, full-time student, you can take out two types of loan: a loan for tuition fees and a maintenance loan to meet living costs. The tuition fees loan does not depend on your household income and is paid straight to the university to cover the full cost. You can borrow all or part of the amount required to cover your fees.

The amount of maintenance loan you are entitled to depends on several factors, including household income, where you live while you're studying, what year of study you are in and what help you get through the maintenance grant (see below).

If you're living away from home, the maximum loan for English students is £5,500 for the academic year (2012–13), although it's more if you're studying in London. The maximum available is less if you're living with your parents during term time. The costs vary depending on which part of the UK you normally live in and are shown in the table below.

Maximum maintenance loan available in 2012–13

Living arrangements during term time	Maximum maintenance loan available in England	Maximum maintenance loan available in Scotland	Maximum maintenance loan available in Wales	Maximum maintenance loan available in Northern Ireland
Living with your parents	£4,375	£4,585	£3,673	£3,750
Living away from home and studying in London	£7,675	£6,690	£6,648	£6,780
Living away from home and studying outside London	£5,500	£5,570	£4,745	£4,840

All figures are taken from the student finance websites listed on page 103.

It is vital to remember when considering student loans that both the tuition fee and living expenses loans are not like loans you would get from a bank. Firstly, interest rates are much lower than for bank loans and so the overall cost of borrowing is very reasonable. Secondly and most importantly, student loans only start being paid back when you have a job that pays over a certain amount. Currently these thresholds are £21,000 per annum for English and Welsh students and £15,795 for Scottish and Northern Irish students. The repayments are then taken directly from your pay packet.

Student grants

The maintenance grant is designed to help home students with accommodation and other living costs incurred while enrolled on a full-time course. These grants don't have to be repaid, but the amount of grant a student receives depends on an assessment made by the local authority based on how much a student's parents earn. A student will only get a full grant if household income is judged to be £25,000 or less. Smaller amounts are available on a sliding scale, but any household with an income above £42,600 will not be eligible for any grant. An idea of the amount of grant awarded is given in the table below.

Amount of maintenance grant available based on family income in 2011–12

Household income	Maintenance grant for 2012–13
Up to £25,000	£3,250
£30,000	£2,341
£35,000	£1,432
£40,000	£523
£42,600	Up to £50
More than £42,600	No grant

Source: www.direct.gov.uk/en/EducationAndLearning/UniversityAndHigher Education/StudentFinance/Typesoffinance/DG_171557

If your application for a maintenance grant is successful, the value of this will be deducted from your maintenance loan.

NHS bursaries

In 2012, NHS bursaries are available for full- and part-time students. To be eligible for such a bursary, a student must qualify as a home student and be on a 'pre-registration health professional training course'. During the first four years of study, dental students are entitled to apply for tuition fee and maintenance loans from Student Finance. From year five onwards, dental students are eligible to apply for a means-tested NHS bursary alongside a reduced student loan to cover maintenance costs. In addition, fees in year five are paid in full by the NHS Student Bursaries scheme. For more information, see the NHS Student Bursaries website (www.nhsbsa.nhs.uk/students).

Scholarships

Certain universities make scholarships available, and these can be a valuable source of income throughout a course. There are some general scholarships as well as ones available only to dentistry students. Details can be obtained from the individual universities, but websites such as www.scholarship-search.org.uk can provide comprehensive lists of available funding.

In addition to this, the armed forces make scholarships available to students wishing to pursue a career in the medical services. These can be particularly lucrative and will often cover tuition fees as well as paying an annual salary for a part of the course. For example, some cadetships will pay all of your tuition fees, plus an annual salary for your last three years of study and a book allowance. Obviously, this route will not appeal to all students, as it guides you into a career in the armed forces. See page 111 for more details.

10 | What career pathways exist for dentists?

Once you have qualified as a dentist, there are a surprising number of different career pathways that can be followed. This chapter looks at the various options that would be open to you, what each of them entails, and some of the potential advantages and disadvantages of each route.

General dental practitioners (GDPs)

Out of the 39,307 registered dentists in the UK, some will run their own dental practices, while others will work in larger practices or groups of practices. Some will carry out NHS work, while others may take only private patients. A large number of dental practices will offer both NHS and private treatment. Private patients have a much wider range of treatment available to them, but they or their dental insurance scheme providers pay the full cost – which is determined by the dentist rather than by the NHS. As a result, charges for private dental work can fluctuate widely across the country. It is estimated that about 1 million people have private dental plans.

Regardless of these differences, most dentists follow a similar path after graduation. During their final year at dental school, students need to consider where they wish to begin their career. The path chosen will vary depending on the individual student's abilities and interests. Many dental schools organise 'going into practice' days for their students, supplementing information available from the BDA.

Students qualifying at a UK dental school must first complete one year of paid, supervised vocational or foundation training (VT/FT) in an approved training practice. During VT, the newly graduated dentists (known as vocational dental practitioners or VDPs) work under supervision in such approved training practices. VDPs are paid by the NHS, and their trainers are also paid an allowance. Any earnings generated by a VDP go to the trainer. Following VT, dentists usually enter an established general practice as an associate or as an assistant.

There is a difference between assistant dentists and associate dentists. Assistant dentists (sometimes known as employed performers) are employed by the practice owner and are paid a salary; associate dentists (sometimes known as performers) are self-employed and are responsible for the treatment that they provide, but work in a practice owned by someone else. The associate dentist buys services from the practice owner, such as nursing or technician support, materials and access to patients, paying the practice owner either a percentage of their earnings or a fixed monthly fee. In some areas, a number of practices prefer to employ assistant dentists. An assistantship provides an opportunity to work as a full member of the practice team but without the uncertainties of a role as an associate.

At a later point in their career, many dentists decide to acquire their own practice. They can do so by buying an existing practice, starting a brand new practice or becoming a partner in an existing practice. Whichever they opt for, it ultimately means they are self-employed and involved in running a small business. In addition to being dentists they are thus also business people and are responsible not only for the treatment that they provide for their own patients but also for the administration of the practice, and the employment of associate dentists if necessary. This element of a career in dentistry can be an attractive proposition, as it allows a love of dentistry and a flair for business to be developed side by side; however, there can be greater stresses and risks associated with following this path.

A very important aspect of a career in dentistry is the ongoing professional development that takes place; a dentist is responsible for structuring and developing their career at their own pace and in the direction they wish. This means that a dentist is always learning and seeking to develop new skills and knowledge in their profession.

Like medical general practitioners, GDPs have the opportunity to form long-term relationships with their patients and provide them with continuing care. This means that a dentist can develop long-term community links and make a real difference to the area where they are based.

Case study 8 illustrates the experience of one dentist through the VT programme.

Case study 8: Dr Neva Patel

Dr Neva Patel completed her degree at King's College London: 'When I qualified, I wasn't sure whether I wanted to become a GDP or work in another field, such as orthodontics or paediatric dentistry. I decided to spend a year in the hospital to gain experience in a range of dental fields.

'Working as a house officer was a very comfortable way of being introduced to dentistry – I saw four to five patients a session, and was able to call on experts if and when the need arose. However, I did not particularly enjoy hospital politics, and I also realised that I did not want a career in research, and so I started my compulsory year's training under a dentist in a dental practice.

'I was very lucky with my trainer, who was extremely helpful and supportive. I enjoyed the year at the practice so much that I stayed on to practise there, and have been there ever since. Among my group of friends who qualified as dentists, I was the only one to stay on at the same practice after VT. I started off gradually, seeing perhaps five to 10 patients a day, so that I could spend time on the treatment. At first, I could take up to an hour on a filling, but I soon became quicker and more confident. The big difference between now and when I first started is that I am not worried about what will come in through the door – I feel that I can cope with anything. The job does have stressful times, of course, particularly when dealing with difficult or aggressive patients. However much you are taught about stress management and dealing with anxious patients at dental school, it cannot prepare you for the real thing.

'Some patients can be aggressive because they are scared. I find that the best way to deal with nervous patients is to explain to them exactly what I am doing at all times. Whenever I use a new instrument, I tell the patient what it is for, and what I will do with it. I explain why I am taking X-rays, and the likely lifetime of the treatment that I am performing. Otherwise, they cannot see what is going on, and can become more frightened. The best part of the job, for me, is when my patients are genuinely pleased with the treatment: I find it very gratifying when new patients are referred by existing ones. I also like the flexibility of the job, and the fact that I can control my hours.

'My position is slightly unusual because I am a salaried dentist. This enables me to spend more time with my patients if they need it, and to devote some time to teaching patients about dental health. I don't have to worry about filling my day to maximise my earnings. It means that there is a limit to what I earn, but it also adds to job satisfaction.'

Hospital and community dentists

Hospital dentistry

Hospital dentistry concentrates on more specialist areas such as orthodontics, restorative dentistry for victims of accidents or illness, paediatric dentistry or oral medicine. As a hospital dentist, the career path is similar to that followed by a doctor: junior, specialty and so on, up to consultant level.

Unlike GDPs, hospital dentists receive a salary. Hospital dentistry is thus possibly less risky, as it is salaried, full-time employment (see also case study 8 above). Hospital dentists generally work as part of a team, have access to specialised diagnostic facilities and work with consultants in other specialisations. Another advantage is that, in the hospital service, there is a prescribed and well-defined career structure and training pathway. However, the hours are not as flexible and time will be spent 'on call', resulting in long working sessions.

Salaried primary care dental service

Some newly qualified dentists prefer to follow a more structured path, and choose to become part of the salaried primary care dental service (SPCDS), which provides dental treatment for a wide range of patients with special needs. As with the hospital service, these posts are salaried and there is a career structure, but this option is less structured than working in the hospital setting. It is possible to carry out your VT in the SPCDS.

Having completed VT, experience is gained as a community clinical dental officer (CCDO), with further opportunity to gain postgraduate qualifications through part-time study. Ambitious CCDOs may wish to become senior dental officers (SDOs), with special responsibilities such as health promotion, epidemiology or treating patients with special needs.

Other careers in dentistry

In addition to the common career paths outlined above, dentists can also find employment in the armed forces and industry. For those with an interest in the academic aspects of dentistry, there are also opportunities for research or teaching in universities; some dentists will opt to become teachers or lecturers in dental schools and involved in research.

Dental bodies corporate (DBCs)

A relatively new development is the increased possibility of working for a body corporate (i.e. a private dental firm), some of which actively recruit dentists from overseas.

The BDA has an advice sheet on working for corporate bodies, which is available to members. By law, DBCs have to be registered with the GDC. This sector is currently on the increase, due to a general move away from NHS dentistry, a growing consumerism among the general public (e.g. wealthier patients demanding top-notch care) and deregulation of the profession, allowing dentists to advertise, thus making company branding possible. A further reason given by the BDA is the belief of venture capitalists, among others, that investment in dentistry will yield attractive returns.

Dentistry in the armed forces

According to the BDA, all three defence forces employ dentists to provide a comprehensive service for personnel, both abroad and in the UK. Dentists hold a commissioned rank and there is a very structured career path to follow. One of the possible benefits of following this route is that financial scholarships may be available during your studies. It is also possible to carry out VT in this sector. For more information on careers in armed forces dentistry, visit the army's website and the Defence Dental Services' website, provided by the Ministry of Defence:

- www.army.mod.uk/army-medical-services/radc/5335.aspx
- www.gov.uk/defence-medical-services#defence-dental-services

Dentistry in industry

Some large manufacturing and engineering companies (for example, oil companies and car manufacturers) offer dental services to their employees. These posts are salaried but the role is equivalent to that of a GDP.

University teaching and research

If you like both teaching and research at university level, there are opportunities in this field. Careers in university dental schools allow you to specialise in a particular aspect of dentistry, which can enable you to pursue research into a specific interest in great depth. University dental teachers will have gained postgraduate qualifications and can progress to become senior lecturers or professors and, if they so wish, get involved with writing teaching materials.

Running a business

Running a dental practice involves all of the skills required in running a business as well as the skills needed to be a dentist. This means that a practice will have to rent or buy a site, employ qualified staff, train them, pay tax and so on. The income of a practice serves to pay the employees, rates and rent. A proportion of the profit is reinvested in the practice for new equipment or new facilities, so that it can continue to offer the best service to its patients. Dentists will be managing a team of people encompassing dental nurses, hygienists, receptionists and others, so good administrative and managerial abilities are needed.

Running a practice can potentially be lucrative, but there are a number of factors that must be considered carefully. These are things such as working long hours, stress and frustrations with the NHS – all of which can be disheartening and unpleasant for a dentist to deal with.

Case study 9: Dr Tom Fraser

Dr Tom Fraser studied at the University of Liverpool. After graduation, he spent a year working in a large NHS practice in Birmingham before joining his father to work in the family practice. He now divides his time between the family practice and a private practice in the Cotswolds that specialises in cosmetic smile enhancements.

'What I find most rewarding about my job is being able to help overcome a patient's anxiety about being treated; this always provides a great degree of satisfaction. I also really enjoy giving patients the confidence to smile! However, as with most professions, there are always challenging aspects of a job that have to be faced on a day-to-day basis. In particular, I find the management of some patients can be very emotionally exhausting. I think it was Lord Winston who said spending a day seeing patients can be draining because you have to give each one a small piece of you; this is certainly true from my experience. On top of the challenges associated with patient care, making sure that administrative tasks are completed can also take up a significant amount of my time and cause some stress.

'In my opinion, one of the most important current issues relating to dentistry is ensuring that all members of the team are adequately trained; it is vitally important that everybody has opportunities to pursue professional development and thereby further their knowledge and skills.

'My tips for aspiring dentists are to work hard to achieve what you want in your career, but at the same time remember the best policy is to be honest and humble at all times.'

The wider team

Being a dentist in any setting is not just about working on your own carrying out dental treatments; a vital part is working within a team made up of numerous different members. The people who work most closely with dentists are dental nurses, dental hygienists and receptionists or administrative staff. The point of mentioning these team members is to raise awareness of some of the important people that you will need to find, employ and train as a practice partner or owner.

Dental nurses

Perhaps the most important person as far as the dentist is concerned is the dental nurse, who plays a key role in any dental practice. Working alongside the dentist, it is the nurse's job to provide a high standard of care for patients and to be the dentist's assistant. They provide skilled supportive care and are able to perform diagnostic tests such as X-rays.

Dental hygienists

The dental hygienist is also a very important part of the dental team. They are licensed dental professionals with a degree or diploma, specialising in preventive dental care and focusing on techniques in oral hygiene. In most cases, the hygienist is employed by a dental practice. Procedures performed by hygienists include cleaning, scaling, radiography and dental sealing.

Receptionists

The first person you will encounter when you telephone or visit a dental practice is the receptionist. The receptionist is there to manage patients' bookings. In practices where there are multiple practitioners, efficient and effective receptionists and administrative staff are crucial to the viability and long-term profit and health of the practice. In taking care of the appointments process and correspondence at a busy practice, they allow dentists more time to focus on their work.

Women in the profession

It was just over a century ago that Lilian Murray (later Lindsay) became the first qualified woman dentist, in 1895. At the end of 2011, 43% of dentists registered with the GDC were women, and according to the BDA this figure is expected to rise to over 50% by the year 2020. In 2011, approximately 57% of new entrants to dental undergraduate courses in the UK were female; in 2012, just over 55% of all applicants were female.

So in just over a century, women have gone from not being represented in the profession at all to acceptance and potential dominance. Dentistry is a good career choice for a woman and, according to a BDA survey, 93% of women dentists responded that their positive career expectations when entering dental school had been fulfilled. Women leaving dental school expect that, if they wish, they will be able to combine a professional career with caring for a family and/or postgraduate study. The primary reasons for women choosing the profession in the survey appeared to be career flexibility, caring for and working with people, and the opportunity to combine practical and intellectual work. Anticipated financial rewards did not seem to be a major factor.

Salaries and wages

According to Prospects Career Planner (www.prospects.ac.uk/dentist_salary.htm) a typical starting salary for a dentist in their first year out of medical school as a VDP is £30,132 (January 2012 figure). This is expected to increase significantly over the career of a dentist, but the amount by which it increases will depend on the career path that a dentist chooses. According to the NHS, in 2009–10 the average gross earnings of a self-employed dentist were £101,700 for a performer-only dentist (one who does not have a contract with a local health body) and £370,900 for a providing-performer dentist (one who has contracts with local health bodies). Before you begin to think about how many Ferraris you could buy when you start earning these amounts, you should be aware that the expenses associated with running a practice (for instance, wages, materials and the practice building) can take approximately 50% of this. Therefore, in 2009–10, after deduction of expenses, the average income was £65,600 for a performer-only dentist and £128,000 for a providing-performer dentist.

A dentist who opts to work in a salaried post in SPCDS can expect to earn between £37,714 and £80,674 (January 2012). Other salaried posts exist in the armed forces and in corporate practices. In NHS hospitals, salaries at the consultant level range from £74,504 to £100,446 (January 2012).

It is not surprising that, in the private sector, dentists will earn on average around the £120,000 to £140,000 mark after expenses. This can, of course, be far greater, depending on the type of dental practice and the amount of work a dentist is prepared to do. For instance, surgical and cosmetic dentistry are two areas that command the high-end costs in the market.

One factor to consider is that, unlike other careers where earnings rise year after year, dentists often reach a peak in their thirties, and their earnings can fall after this as they become older, slower and less inclined to work long hours.

Case study 10: Dr George Mitchell

Dr George Mitchell qualified as a dental surgeon from Birmingham Dental School in 1976. He has worked at several dental practices and was a part-time clinical assistant dental surgeon at West Heath Hospital (treating the elderly) for 18 years. His own practice carries out private treatment on adults. NHS treatment is provided for children.

'I'm a GDP, so I carry out a wide range of treatments for my patients, but I have a particular interest in the areas of restorative dentistry, cosmetic dentistry and the dental care of the elderly. There is a long history of dentistry in my family; both my father and grandfather were dentists so my practice is long established.

'There are great opportunities for professional development as a dentist and continually developing knowledge and skills by attending courses and keeping up to date with the latest developments. These are enjoyable elements of the profession. I also really enjoy the interaction with people that the job affords; meeting patients and colleagues and interacting with technicians and dental companies is particularly rewarding.

'There are a great deal of challenges involved in being a dentist: I have to ensure that I provide an excellent level of service for my patients at an affordable price while at the same time keeping costs under control so that I can make a reasonable income. It is also vital to keep up with the ever-changing advances in procedures and equipment.

'Aspiring dentists should realise that when following this vocation it helps if you are hard-working and like helping people; this is not a job that you should do just because of the money. It is also important to understand that running a practice requires a range of skills, as it is really like running a small business.'

Graduate prospects

In a recent study, the Office for National Statistics found that at the end of 2011, 18.9% of graduates who had graduated in the past two years were out of work (www.ons.gov.uk/ons/dcp171776_259049.pdf). With such high levels of graduate unemployment it is worth considering whether a dentistry degree will be an asset or a liability in the job market of the future, and what the prospects are for successfully entering employment following the completion of your dental degree and training.

The *Guardian*'s online university guide (www.guardian.co.uk/education/universityguide) gives data on the number of graduates from each dental school being employed six months after graduation. The general picture here is that the job market for dentists remains buoyant and there is still strong demand, and indeed a very high probability of being employed soon after finishing your education. The percentage of graduates in employment after six months ranges from 97% to 100%, with an average employment rate of 99.6%. This is 1% higher than in 2009, so job prospects remain outstanding, in spite of the difficult economic climate. Even more reassuring is that there are 10 dental schools reporting a 100% success rate; a figure that has doubled since 2009. This is an amazing statistic, considering the current state of the graduate jobs market.

At this point in time and for the foreseeable future, it seems that a dentistry degree will represent a solid investment and lead to excellent job prospects following graduation. At a time when so many graduates are struggling to find work, this potentially makes studying dentistry an even more attractive proposition than it already was.

11| Further information

Further reading

There is a wealth of information available both on the internet and beyond. Try to keep up to date with some of the key developments as this will give you an excellent overview of what is happening in the world of dentistry.

An essential starting point is the BDA's website (www.bda.org). This carries careers information for prospective dentists as well as press releases and discussion of topical issues. The BDA's website for dental patients (www.bdasmile.org) is also useful.

The BDA has its own museum, the BDA Dental Museum, which gives an interesting historical overview of dentistry; details can be found at www.bda.org/museum. Some other useful websites are www.dentistry.co.uk, www.dentalhealth.org, www.gdc-uk.org and www.3dmouth.org. These all have a wealth of factual information and details of current affairs relating to dentistry and as such are worth a regular look. www.thestudentroom.co.uk is a chat room for potential students and has a number of interesting discussions relating to dental admissions; however, double check any information you receive from here as it may not always be reliable.

The BDA publishes a journal for dentists, the *British Dental Journal* (www.nature.com/bdj). The journal is aimed at practising dentists and can be very technical, although it does give very good short summaries of some of the most relevant hot topics. The International Society for Fluoride Research publishes its own journal called *Fluoride*. Some articles from the journal are available on the society's website (www.fluorideresearch.org).

To keep up to date with dentistry and dental issues in the UK, the *Independent*, the *Guardian*, the *Daily Telegraph* and *The Times* all carry regular health reporting and have health sections once a week. Another source of dental news is the website www.topix.net/business/dental, which covers topical dentistry stories from the UK and worldwide.

For summaries of course information and academic requirements, a useful reference point is *HEAP 2014 University Degree Course Offers*, written by Brian Heap and published by Trotman (www.trotman.co.uk), or *The UCAS Guide to Getting into University and College* (www. ucasbooks.co.uk).

Tables

The tables on the next few pages will give you more information about dental school applications, required grades and typical offers so that you have a clear idea of what each school expects from its applicants.

- **Table 1** shows the number of applicants to dental school over four years, from 2006 to 2011, through UCAS.
- **Table 2** presents dental school admissions policies for 2013 entry.
- **Table 3** presents the statistics for dental school applications in 2011.
- **Table 4** shows you typical interview styles and lengths for each dental school and how many people will be on the panel for 2013 entry.
- **Table 5** shows typical costs for a range of dental procedures for reference.
- **Table 6** shows what requirements are needed for students wishing to apply to pre-dental courses in 2013.
- **Table 7** has the requirements for graduate entry to dental school in 2013.

Table 1 Applicants through UCAS to dentistry by the October deadline – 2006–11

Year	Total applicants	Male – UK	Female – UK	Male – EU	Female – EU	Male – non-EU	Female – non-EU
2006	2,911	1,154	1,310	74	121	111	141
2007	3,114	1,224	1,463	83	114	106	124
2008	2,995	1,209	1,388	70	112	80	136
2009	3,304	1,287	1,558	70	120	93	176
2010	3,720	1,438	1,727	95	178	117	165
2011	3,197	1,273	1,451	61	127	102	183
Percentage change 2006–11	+9.8%	+10.3%	+10.8%	–17.6%	+5.0%	–8.1%	+29.8%
Percentage change 2010–11	–14.1%	–11.5%	–16.0%	–35.8%	–28.7%	–12.8%	+10.9%

Information extracted from www.ucas.ac.uk/about_us/stat_services/stats_online/data_tables.

Table 2 Dental school admissions policies – 2013 entry

University	Standard offer	GCSE requirements	Approximate percentage of applicants interviewed	Retakes considered?	Retake offer	Sciences preferred	UKCAT policy
Belfast	AAA + A at AS	Mathematics and either Physics or Double Science if not offered at AS or A level. Best 9 scored: 4 points per A*, 3 points per A	–	Yes – if applied to Queen's at first attempt, held an offer as their first choice and achieved AAB at first sitting	–	Chemistry plus at least one other from Biology/ Human Biology, Mathematics and Physics. Biology to AS grade B or above if not offered at A level	Required
Birmingham	AAA + A/B at AS	Chemistry and Biology at A*A*, or Double Science at A*A*. Mathematics and English Language at A	40%	No	–	Chemistry and Biology/ Human Biology	Not required
Bristol	AAA	Minimum of 5 at A*/A, including English Language, Mathematics and 2 sciences	30%	No	–	Chemistry and one other lab-based science (preferably Biology). Grade A in AS Biology if not offered at A level	Not required
Cardiff	AAA	English Language, Mathematics, Science and Additional Science all at B (or single science subjects – Biology, Chemistry and Physics – with 2 at B)	20%	No	–	Biology and Chemistry at grade A, but no preference on the third subject (Critical Thinking and General Studies are excluded)	Required

Dundee	AAA	English Language at C, plus one from Chemistry, Physics and Mathematics (if not taken at A level) at B	45%	No	–	Biology and two from Chemistry, Physics and Mathematics	Required
Glasgow	AAB (with at least BBB at first sitting at end of AS level)	7 at grade B or above, including English Language and Literature and Physics and/or Mathematics	50%	Yes – if applied previously and held a conditional offer which was missed by a narrow margin	AAA	Human Biology or Biology at grade A plus Chemistry at grade A	Required
King's	AAA + A at AS	At least B in English Literature and Mathematics if not offered at AS or A level	40%	No	–	Biology and Chemistry, with at least one at A level and the other at AS level	Required
Leeds	AAA	Minimum of 6, including English, Mathematics, Chemistry and Biology (or Double Science), with minimum C in both English and Mathematics at GCSE or equivalent	30%	Yes	AAA	Biology and Chemistry	Not required
Liverpool	AAA	Minimum of 7 at A, with Mathematics and English Language at A or above	45%	No	–	Biology and Chemistry	Not required
Manchester	AAA + B at AS	6 at a minimum of A (including Double Science or Physics, Chemistry and Biology) and B or above in English Language and Mathematics	25%	Yes – minimum CCC at first sitting	A*AA	Biology and Chemistry	Required

Table 2 Continued

University	Standard offer	GCSE requirements	Approximate percentage of applicants interviewed	Retakes considered?	Retake offer	Sciences preferred	UKCAT policy
Newcastle	AAA	5 at A or above, including Biology and Chemistry or Double Science	35%	Yes – if held conditional offer in previous cycle, had Newcastle as their first choice, but failed to meet the terms of the offer	AAA	Biology and Chemistry	Required
Plymouth	AAA + C at AS	English Language, Mathematics and either Single and Additional Science or Biology and Chemistry at A–C	–	Yes – if achieved ABB at first sitting	–	–	Not required
Queen Mary	AAA + B at AS	AAABBB or above (in any order), including Biology (or Human Biology), Chemistry (or Double Science), English Language and Mathematics (or Additional Mathematics or Statistics)	40%	No	–	Biology and Chemistry at AS level plus at least one at A level	Required
Sheffield	AAA	6 at A, including Mathematics, English Language and Science	25%	Yes	AAA	Biology and Chemistry	Required

All information taken from www.ucas.ac.uk and from individual university websites.

Table 3 Dental school application statistics – an example of the number of applicants to dental schools in 2011

University	Applications	Interviews	Offers	Accepted	Clearing	Graduates	Overseas students	Resits
Belfast	179	11	70	46	1	4	0	8
Birmingham	751	350	140	75	0	3 to 5	0	0
Bristol	824	220	100	75	0	Not available	4	0
Cardiff	850	200	165	83	0	4	5	0
Dundee	369	177	144	66	0	3	7	0
Glasgow	550	258	161	95	2	14	3	7
King's	1,468	576	236	167	0	25	12	0
Leeds	1,352	386	202	81	0	2	3	5
Liverpool	970	450	150	62	0	9	2	0
Manchester	966	230	153	75	0	6	4	4
Newcastle	700	231	126	78	0	14	7	4
Queen Mary	596	236	135	61	0	2	8	0
Sheffield	896	Approx. 200	120	75	6	2	4	Not available

All information obtained individually from the admissions team of each dental school.

Table 4 Typical interviews – 2013 entry

University	Type of interview	Number on panel	Other information
Belfast	Multiple mini interviews designed to test a range of non-cognitive skills	Each mini interview is conducted by a pair of interviewers	Scores at interview are used to rank applicants. Offers are made to the highest ranking interviewees
Birmingham	Panel interview	2/3	Approximately 15 minutes long
Bristol	Multiple mini interviews conducted by a number of staff	n/a	During the interviews, students will visit 10 stations spending 7 minutes at each. Each station will have a task that the applicants will complete before moving on to the next
Cardiff	Multiple mini interviews	Most stations have one interviewer; two stations have two interviewers	None
Dundee	Multiple mini interviews, including five traditional format interviews and five practical and hands-on interviews	n/a	Consists of 10 7-minute interviews, with the whole process lasting 70 minutes
Glasgow	Multiple mini interviews	n/a	None
King's	Multiple mini interviews	One or two at each station	Interviewees circulate from one timed station to another. At each station interviewers ask structured questions and mark the responses to the questions independently
Leeds	Multiple mini interviews	n/a	None
Liverpool	Multiple mini interviews	n/a	None

Manchester	Panel interview	2/3		The panel comprises two practising clinicians. A third member may be present to act as the chair
Newcastle	Panel interview	2		The panel comprises members of academic staff, at least one of whom will be a clinician
Plymouth	Panel interview	3/4		The panel can comprise a clinician, a non-clinical academic, a healthcare professional and a lay community member
Queen Mary	Panel interview	3		None
Sheffield	Panel interview	3		The panel comprises a clinical member of staff, an academic member of staff and a senior dental student

Table 5 Dental procedure costs

Band 1 course of treatment: £17.50

- Clinical examination, case assessment and report
- Orthodontic case assessment and report
- Advice, dental charting, diagnosis and treatment planning
- Radiographic examination, including panoral and lateral headplates, and radiological report
- Study casts including in association with occlusal analysis
- Colour photographs
- Instruction in the prevention of dental and oral disease including dietary advice and dental hygiene instruction
- Surface application as primary preventive measures of sealants and topical fluoride preparations
- Scaling, polishing and marginal correction of fillings
- Taking material for pathological examination
- Adjustments to and easing of dentures or orthodontic appliances
- Treatment of sensitive cementum

Band 2 course of treatment: £48.00

- Non-surgical periodontal treatment including rootplaning, deep scaling, irrigation of periodontal pockets and subgingival curettage and all necessary scaling and polishing

- Surgical periodontal treatment, including gingivectomy, gingivoplasty or removal of an operculum
- Surgical periodontal treatment, including raising and replacement of a mucoperiosteal flap, curettage, root planing and bone resection
- Free gingival grafts
- Permanent fillings in amalgam, composite resin, synthetic resin, glass ionomer, compomers, silicate or silico-phosphate, including acid etch retention
- Sealant restorations
- Endodontic treatment of permanent or retained deciduous teeth
- Pulpotomy
- Apicectomy
- Extraction of teeth
- Transplantation of teeth
- Oral surgery including surgical removal of cyst, buried root, unerupted tooth, impacted tooth or exostosed tooth and alveolectomy
- Soft tissue surgery in relation to the buccal cavity and lips
- Frenectomy, frenuloplasty and frenotomy
- Relining and rebasing dentures including soft linings
- Addition of tooth, clasp, labial or buccal flange to dentures
- Splints (other than laboratory-made splints) in relation to periodontally compromised teeth and in connection with external trauma
- Bite-raising appliances (other than laboratory-made appliances)

Band 3 course of treatment: £209.00

- Laboratory-made porcelain or composite veneers, including acid etch retention
- Inlays, pinlays, onlays and palatal veneers, in alloys containing 60% or more fine gold, porcelain, composite resin and ceramics
- Crowns including any pin or post aids to retention:
  - full or three-quarter crown cast in alloys containing not less than 33⅓% fine gold or platinum or palladium
  - full or jacket crown cast in alloys containing stainless steel or cobalt chromium or nickel chromium
  - crown in porcelain, synthetic resin and other non-metallic crowns
  - full or jacket crowns in alloys containing not less than 33⅓% fine gold or platinum or palladium, or alloys containing stainless steel or cobalt chromium or nickel chromium, with thermally bonded porcelain
  - jacket crown thermally bonded to wrought platinum coping
  - prefabricated full or jacket crown, including any pin or post retention
- Bridges including any pin or post aids to retention:
  - bridges in alloys containing 60% or more fine gold with or without thermally bonded facings
  - bridges cast in alloys containing stainless steel, cobalt chromium or nickel chromium, with or without thermally bonded facings
  - acid etch retained bridges
  - bridges in other materials
  - provision of full (completed) or partial dentures, overdentures and obturators in synthetic resin or metal or both synthetic resin and metal, including any cast or wrought metal components or aids to retention
  - orthodontic treatment and appliances
  - other custom-made applications excluding sports guards

Source: Reprinted with kind permission from NHS Choices

Table 6 Pre-dental course entry requirements – 2013 entry

University	Standard offer	GCSE requirements	A level subject requirements	UKCAT policy
Cardiff	AAA	English Language and Mathematics at B, plus 2 from Biology, Chemistry and Physics at B or above. Science and Additional Science at B or above also acceptable	AAA grades required with no more than 1 coming from Biology, Chemistry or Physics	Required
Dundee	AAA	English Language and preferably Biology	No more than 1 science A level	Required
Manchester	AAA + B at AS	At least 7 subjects including Chemistry, Biology, Physics (or Double Science), Mathematics and English Language. At least 5 subjects must be at a minimum of grade A with English Language at a minimum of grade B	3 arts subjects or 2 arts subjects and 1 science subject, including grade B in one AS subject	Required

Note: The pre-dental course at Bristol was discontinued in September 2012.

Table 7 Entry requirements for graduate courses – 2013 entry

University	Pre-degree requirements	Degree requirements	Interview	UKCAT policy
Aberdeen	None	2.i in a medical science subject or a MBChB	Yes	Required
King's	None	At least 2.i in a biomedically related or health professional subject or a 2.ii in a biomedically related or health professional subject with a postgraduate degree (with at least a merit)	Yes	Required
Liverpool	3 A levels at C or above, 2 of which must be sciences (Geography and Sociology are not acceptable). One of the sciences must be Biology or Chemistry; if either Biology or Chemistry is not offered at A level it must be offered at AS level with B or above. GCSE Mathematics and English Language at C or above. Good performance at either A levels (minimum 2 grade As) or GCSEs (minimum 5 grade As).	2.i or above in a biomedical sciences subject or a MBChB from an approved institution	Yes	Not required
University of Central Lancashire (UCLan)	3 A levels at C or above, including 2 from Biology, Chemistry, Physics and Mathematics. GCSE Mathematics and English Language at B.	2.i in a biomedical subject	Yes	Not required

Postgraduate deaneries in the UK

Defence

Group Captain Dermot McCarthy
Defence Postgraduate Dental Dean

Defence Postgraduate Medical Deanery
DMS Whittington
Whittington Barracks
Lichfield WS14 9PY
Website: www.gov.uk/defence-medical-services#defence-dental-services

Eastern

Professor Simon Gregory
Postgraduate Dean

East of England Multi-Professional Deanery
CPC1
Capital Park
Fulbourn
Cambridge CB21 5XE
Website: www.eoedeanery.nhs.uk/page.php?area_id=11
Tel: 01223 743 300
Fax: 01223 743 301

London

Elizabeth Jones
Dean of Postgraduate Dentistry

Dental Department
LPMDE
London Deanery
Stewart House
32 Russell Square
London WC1B 5DN
Website: www.londondeanery.ac.uk
Tel: 020 7866 3100

Mersey

Brian Grieveson
Dean of Postgraduate Dental Education and Training

Mersey Deanery
Regatta Place
Brunswick Business Park

Summers Road
Liverpool L3 4BL
Website: www.merseydeanery.nhs.uk
Tel: 0151 285 4700/4701
Fax: 0151 285 4703

North

Chris Gray
Postgraduate Dental Dean

Northern Deanery
Waterfront 4
Goldcrest Way
Newburn Riverside
Newcastle upon Tyne NE15 8NY
Website: www.northerndeanery.nhs.uk/NorthernDeanery
Tel: 0191 210 6400 (main switchboard)
Fax: 0191 210 6401 (reception)

North West

Nicholas Taylor
Director of Postgraduate Dental Education

North Western Deanery
Three Piccadilly Place
Manchester M1 3BN
Website: www.nwpgmd.nhs.uk
Tel: 0845 050 0194 (main switchboard)
Fax: 0161 625 7502

Northern Ireland

David Hussey
Postgraduate Dental Dean

NIMDTA
Beechill House
42 Beechill Road
Belfast BT8 7RL
Website: www.nimdta.gov.uk
Tel: 028 9040 0000

Oxford

Helen Falcon
Postgraduate Dental Dean

Oxford Postgraduate Medical and Dental Education
Oxford Deanery
The Triangle
Roosevelt Drive
Headington
Oxford OX3 7XP
Website: www.oxforddeanery.nhs.uk
Tel: 01865 740601
Fax: 01865 740636

Scotland

Dr David Felix
Postgraduate Dental Dean

NHS Education for Scotland
Westport 102
West Port
Edinburgh EH39DN
Website: www.nes.scot.nhs.uk
Tel: 0131 656 3200
Fax: 0131 656 3201

South

Professor Stephen Lambert-Humble
Dean of Postgraduate Dentistry

The Dental Department
KSS Postgraduate Deanery
7 Bermondsey Street
London SE1 2DD
Website: http://kssdeanery.org/dental
Tel: 020 7415 3400

South West

Alasdair Miller
Regional Postgraduate Dental Dean

University of Bristol
Regional Dental Postgraduate Department
Bristol Dental Hospital
Lower Maudlin Street
Bristol BS1 2LY
Website: www.bristol.ac.uk/dentalpg
Tel: 0117 342 4524
Fax: 0117 342 4526

South Yorkshire/East Midlands

Chris Franklin
Postgraduate Dental Dean

Regional Postgraduate Dental Education Office
Don Valley House
Savile Street East
Sheffield S4 7UQ
Website: www.postgraddentalsyem.co.uk
Tel: 0114 226 4454
Fax: 0114 226 4468

Wales

Derek Gallen
Head of School and Dean

Wales Deanery
1st, 8th & 9th Floors
Neuadd Meirionnydd
Heath Park
Cardiff CF14 4YS
Website: www.walesdeanery.org/dentistry
Tel: 029 20687294

Wessex

Helen Falcon
Postgraduate Dental Dean

Wessex Deanery
Southern House
Otterbourne
Winchester SO21 2RU
Website: www.wessexdeanery.nhs.uk
Tel: 01962 718400
Fax: 01962 718401

West Midlands

Karen Elley
Postgraduate Dental Dean

NHS West Midlands
St Chad's Court
213 Hagley Road
Edgbaston B16 9RG

Website: www.westmidlandsdeanery.nhs.uk/Dentistry.aspx
Tel: 0121 695 2222
Fax: 0121 695 2578

Yorkshire

Paul Cook
Regional Postgraduate Dental Dean

Department for NHS Postgraduate Medical and Dental Education
Willow Terrace Road
University of Leeds
Leeds LS2 9JT
Website: www.yorksandhumberdeanery.nhs.uk/dentistry
Tel: 0113 3431557

Organisations

British Dental Association
64 Wimpole Street
London W1G 8YS
Website: www.bda.org
Tel: 020 7935 0875

British Fluoridation Society
PO Box 18
Uppermill
Oldham OL3 6WU
Website: www.bfsweb.org
Tel: 01457 238507

British Medical Association
BMA House
Tavistock Square
London WC1H 9JP
Website: www.bma.org.uk
Tel: 020 7387 4499

General Dental Council
37 Wimpole Street
London W1G 8DQ
Website: www.gdc-uk.org
Tel: 0845 222 4141

Dental schools

University of Aberdeen

Admissions Tutor: Dr Christine Kay
Admissions Secretary: Ms Emma Dunlop

School of Medicine and Dentistry
3rd Floor
Polwarth Building
Foresterhill
Aberdeen AB25 2ZD
Website: www.abdn.ac.uk/medicine-dentistry/medical-dental/
programmes/dentistry
Tel: 01224 437923

University of Birmingham

Admissions Tutor: Mr K Coomar
Admission Secretary: Miss Francis Dean

The School of Dentistry
University of Birmingham
St Chad's Queensway
Birmingham B4 6NN
Website: www.birmingham.ac.uk/schools/dentistry
Tel: 0121 466 5572
Fax: 0121 466 5451

University of Bristol

Admissions Tutor: Dr Michele Barbour
Admission Secretary: Ms Geraldine Vines

School of Oral and Dental Sciences
Lower Maudlin Street
Bristol BS1 2LY
Website: www.bristol.ac.uk/dental
Tel: 0117 923 0000

Cardiff University

Admissions Tutor: Dr Robert McAndrew
Admissions Officer: Mrs Victoria Ocock

Cardiff University
Heath Park

Cardiff CF14 4XY
Website: www.cardiff.ac.uk/dentl/
Tel: 029 2074 2470

University of Central Lancashire

Senior Administrative Assistant: Tracy Farrell

Preston PR1 2HE
Website: www.uclan.ac.uk/schools/dentistry
Tel: 01772 895900

University of Dundee

Admissions Tutor: Ms Fiona Stewart
Information Assistant: Miss Lyn Mitchell

Dundee Dental School
University of Dundee
Park Place
Dundee DD1 4HN
Website: http://dentistry/dundee.ac.uk
Tel: 01382 660111

University of Glasgow

Admissions Tutor: Dr Christine Goodall
Admission Secretary: Miss Rona Miller

Glasgow Dental Hospital and School
378 Sauchiehall Street
Glasgow G2 3JZ
Website: www.gla.ac.uk/schools/dental
Tel: 0141 211 9600
Fax: 0141 331 2798

King's College London

Admissions Tutor: Dr Lyndon Cabot
Admission Assistant: Ms Lisa Frain

Health Schools Admissions Centre
King's College London
1st Floor, Hodgkin Building
London Bridge
London SE1 1UL
Website: www.kcl.ac.uk/dentistry
Tel: 020 7848 6512

University of Leeds

Admissions Tutor: Cath Potter

School of Dentistry
Leeds Dental Institute
Clarendon Way
Leeds LS2 9LU
Website: www.dentistry.leeds.ac.uk/?page_id=50
Tel: 0113 343 6199

University of Liverpool

Admissions Tutor: Dr Tony Preston
Admission Secretary: Miss Abigail Watkins

School of Dentistry
Liverpool University Dental Hospital
Pembroke Place
Liverpool L3 5PS
Website: www.liv.ac.uk/dentistry
Tel: 0151 706 5298

University of Manchester

Admissions Tutor: Dr Anthony Mellor
Admission Secretary: Ms Teresa Smith

School of Dentistry
The University of Manchester
Higher Cambridge Street
Manchester M15 6FH
Website: www.dentistry.manchester.ac.uk
Tel: 0161 306 0239

Newcastle University

Admissions Tutor: Dr David Brown
School Administrator: Ms Michelle Smith

School of Dental Sciences
Newcastle University
Framlington Place
Newcastle upon Tyne NE2 4BW
Website: www.ncl.ac.uk/dental
Tel: 0191 222 8347
Fax: 0191 222 6137

Plymouth University Peninsula Schools of Medicine and Dentistry

Senior Admissions Coordinator: Ms Debbie Coach

Peninsula College of Medicine and Dentistry
John Bull Building
Tamar Science Park
Research Way
Plymouth PL6 8BU
Website: www1.plymouth.ac.uk/peninsula/dentistry
Tel: 01752 437333

Queen Mary (Barts and The London School of Medicine and Dentistry)

Admissions Tutor: Professor Kim Piper
Admission Secretary: Natasha Chapel

Barts and The London School of Medicine and Dentistry
Queen Mary University of London
Turner Street
London E1 2AD
Website: www.dentistry.qmul.ac.uk
Tel: 020 7882 2240

Queen's University Belfast

Admissions Tutor: Mrs Dwyer

Centre for Dental Education
Grosvenor Road
Royal Victoria Hospital
Belfast BT12 6BP
Website: www.qub.ac.uk/schools/mdbs/dentistry
Tel: 028 9063 2733
Fax: 028 9043 8861

University of Sheffield

Admissions Tutor: Mr Duncan Wood
Admission Secretary: Mrs Amanda Okrasa

The School of Clinical Dentistry
University of Sheffield
19 Claremont Crescent
Sheffield S10 2TA
Website: www.sheffield.ac.uk/dentalschool
Tel: 0114 271 7801

Glossary

Assistant dentists
Dentists who are employed by the practice owner and are paid a salary.

Associate dentists
Dentists who are self-employed and are responsible for the treatment that they provide, but work in a practice owned by someone else.

Bachelor of Dental Surgery (BDS)
The degree you will be awarded from most universities upon completion of your dental degree.

BChD
The same as BDS, but the Latin equivalent.

British Dental Association (BDA)
A professional association and trade union for dentists in the United Kingdom.

Clearing
The system whereby students can gain entry to a university course in the period after results are released if they have not achieved the required grades.

Community Clinical Dental Officer (CCDO)
A position within the salaried primary care dental service.

Continuous professional development (CPD)
The ongoing training that a dentist must complete throughout their career. A dentist must complete a specified amount each year.

Endodontics
A dental specialism related to the health of the tooth root and its surrounding tissue.

Fluoride
A group of inorganic fluorine-containing compounds found in water supplies and toothpastes which reduce tooth decay.

General dental practitioner (GDP)
A dentist who provides general dental care to the public either privately or through the NHS.

IELTS
The International English Language Testing System. Students who do not have English as their first language must reach a certain IELTS level in order to gain entry to study dentistry.

Intercalated BSc
At some universities it is possible to take an additional year to complete an intercalated degree. This results in obtaining an extra BSc in addition to the BDS qualification you will receive at the end of the dentistry course.

Multiple mini interviews (MMIs)
An alternative interview format that requires interviewees to move between numerous stations to answer questions.

Orthodontics
A dental specialism involved with the treatment of improper bites.

Overseas Registration Exam (ORE)
Students who complete a dental degree outside the European Economic Area (EEA) are required to complete this exam prior to becoming a registered dentist in this country.

Paediatric dentistry
A specialism related to working with children.

Periodontics
A specialism dealing with the supporting structures of teeth.

Problem-based learning (PBL)
A style of teaching used by some dental schools that relies heavily on independent study.

Prosthodontics
A dental specialism dealing with the replacement of hard and soft tissues using crowns, bridges, dentures and implants.

Salaried Primary Care Dental Service (SPCDS)
The service in the UK that is currently responsible for the treatment of people with special medical or social needs, such as complex medical problems, disabilities or mental health problems, who are unable to be treated by general dental practitioners (GDPs).

Self-directed learning

A style of learning where the student takes responsibility for their direction of study and the study they undertake.

UCAS

The Universities and Colleges Admissions Service. Your application will be made through this service.

The United Kingdom Clinical Aptitude Test (UKCAT)

A pre-admissions test used by most dental schools to distinguish between applicants.

Vocational dental practitioners (VDP)

Graduate dentists who are undertaking their vocational training are known as VDPs.

Vocational training (VT)

The one-year period of training carried out by dentists following graduation.